Y0-CAS-689

Chasing Dragonflies

Life and Care in Aging

Lauren Smerglia Seifert, Ph.D

 CLOVE PRESS LTD, Cuyahoga Falls, OH

I respectfully acknowledge the many authors I have cited and/or quoted. If there are any errors regarding permission to cite those works, or if there are any mistakes in the references, please let me know. I will plan to correct them in a later edition.

Neither the author of this book, nor its publishers intend this book as specific, professional consultation. Readers are cautioned that their own circumstances might require consultation with qualified professionals—which this book does not stand in lieu of.

Publisher's Cataloging-in-Publication
(Provided by Quality Books, Inc.)

Seifert, Lauren Smerglia.
   Chasing dragonflies : life and care in aging / Lauren Smerglia Seifert.
      p. cm.
   Includes bibliographical references and index.
   LCCN 2006909814
   ISBN-13: 978-0-9791023-0-1
   ISBN-10: 0-9791023-0-8

   1. Older people--Care. 2. Dementia--Patients--Care. 3. Aging. 4. Quality of life. I. Title.

HV1451.S454 2007   362.6
                          QBI06-600546

Dedication

For Toby, Mom, and Dad,
Who always knew I could:
Thanks for waiting for me to recognize it,
too.

Special gratitude to Neal Johnson, my
graduate mentor and a wonderful role model.

Special thanks and love to all my family:
my two sibs, my in-law sibs, my beautiful
nieces and nephews, and my wonderful
in-law mom and dad.
Thanks, also, to Mindy & Jon: students-
turned-friends.

L.E.O.
Love Each Other.

Contents

Chapters

Additional Resources

Foreword

The deep green of a mountain-side. Appalachian slopes in July.

I chased spice-bush swallowtails, while my parents redirected our attention to the house where Dad had been born. I was addicted to the breezes....and to the insects. It's a paradox that I became a research psychologist, because I'm truly infatuated with flying bugs: luna moths, monarch butterflies, shimmering dragonflies. At night, it was the lightning bugs. In shady spots, it was the root-boring beetles, which would shock us as they took off from blades of grass. It defied everyday physics. They were so dense. How could they fly?

I think human life is like a wild chase, but it's not so much a goose-chase, as it is a fantastic adventure. We scamper after our dreams and ideals. I think of dragonflies. They are exquisite. They glimmer—fleeting streaks of blue, green, purple, and pink—across ponds, over pools, around reeds. In this volume, I celebrate human life as that quest on a sunny afternoon we've spent chasing dragonflies.

Lauren S. Seifert
September, 2006

Fireflies sprinkle the grass,
At dusk,
With Spring's afterthoughts.

I find you on a white porch—
Azure dress against
Sky of same.

You fold me into your lap.
We pitch,
Like a small boat
On a calm sea,
With sails down,
Forward and Back
Until sleep.

And then,
I am tucked against you.
No more daylight.
No more bright sky.
No more fireflies.
Just happy dreams of us.

--for Grandma at 80
with much love, from Lauren

1

An Introduction to Life and Care in Aging

Four faces leaning forward into a card game: At a dining room table, they tease and laugh. Hands hold cards—fanned out and propped up by elbows on the table. Someone chides, "We're gonna be here all night at this rate. Play your hand already!" The taunted player winks and asks, "Oh, is it *my* turn?" And the other players chuckle.

We live our lives by trying to make meaning. Time with friends or family; a vacation to a beautiful destination; workdays devoted to a professional life: They are the minutes, hours, days, and years of our construction. We make plans and we try to build a meaningful life.

Sitting down to supper conversation about what everyone did that day can be an opportunity to connect. Sometimes, the day's tasks are still going on and dinner is missed—because of a piano lesson, a basketball game, or an evening meeting. When we give our time: to sit down and enjoy our loved ones; to console a friend in tears; to play with a child or a grandchild; to take a walk with a neighbor; to consult a confidant by phone; or to eat a delicious meal—with interesting talk about sports, politics, our kids' report cards, or an upcoming celebration—we are making meaning. *When we donate energy, time, and personal resources in ways that are valued by us and by others, then we can work to improve the quality of human life.*

On a Friday night, my husband and I played cards with my brother and his wife. We laughed and carried on with silly chatter about this-and-that. We munched snacks, dealt cards, and teased each other. We were having fun, and as we did so, it struck me that we are just like the "bridge ladies". They are four women I know who meet each Tuesday evening (and sometimes other nights) to play cards after supper. They tease and laugh. They chitchat about food, the weather, their families, and anything else that comes to mind. They do all of this and more at the long-term care facility where they live.

Their actions are the same as mine: playing a game with friends/family on a pleasant evening. Nevertheless, the bridge ladies' game of cards might seem less important. I can hop into my car and run to the store for more pop and chips. They cannot. My card game is a diversion of leisure from stress. It rejuvenates me for the next week of work, family crises, driving here and there, and meal preparation. Theirs is not. Or is it? What purpose does the card game play in the life of a bridge lady?

We all seem to suffer from the same delusion that *our own days* mean something more than other people's do.[1] We are validated by our racing around, our shuffling papers, our drawing-up plans, our bathing children, and our folding laundry. We have decided which activities mean something and which ones do not. Like Raskolnikov in Dostoyoevsky's famous novel,[2] we engage in a perpetual game of judgment about the relative values of ourselves and others. When we drive too fast, it is because *we must* get to an appointment on time. When others drive too fast and cut us off in traffic, it is because *they are* rude and obnoxious. If I talk too loudly at a movie, it's because I'm having fun with friends, but when a stranger does the same thing, it's because s/he is inconsiderate and idiotic.

How do we arrive at the assessment that values our card game but considers theirs trivial? Why is it so easy to dismiss their behaviors and elevate our own to significance? An individual's sense of meaning is, in part, tied to his/her *attributions*. These are the judgments we make about the causes of people's behavior. In the examples I gave above—of rambunctious road-running and movie mayhem—the common theme is a tendency to excuse one's own bad behaviors, while holding others personally accountable for theirs. *We attribute our own misbehavior to circumstances, but for others we assume a personality flaw is the cause.* These are the foundation of what scientists call "fundamental attribution errors".[3]

A centuries-old expression goes something like: "Whatever you believe, it is so." In the field of sociology, it is called the Thomas Theorem (or the "Thomas Dictum"; Thomas & Thomas, 1928) and paraphrased: whatever one believes, it is 'real in all its consequences'. So it goes that people attribute more meaning to one thing than to another. They believe one thing, but not another, and their actions reflect their beliefs. This reality of belief is played out in fundamental attribution errors every day. Our attribution errors become crystallized when we enact the Thomas Dictum: that is, when we treat our attributions as reality.

We make personal judgments and then proceed to treat them as facts. When we believe, in one moment, that we are worth more than everyone else, then we act as if it were true. If I am late for an appointment, it is because I am over-worked and, after all, I'm doing the best I can—considering all I have to juggle in my hectic life. But when someone is late to meet with me, then s/he is ill-mannered and uncaring. I have turned my internal reality (that my day is worth more) into an error in judgment about someone else. I excuse my own behavior and expect others to do so, because: "I'm a decent person and I didn't mean to make a mess out of everything!" At the same time, I refuse to forgive others for their mistakes, because my attributions tell me that: "They did it on purpose, and they are stupid!"

You can arm yourself with an array of derogatory adjectives to suit all your needs for "rationalized dislike" of another person, e.g., rude, conniving, thoughtless, careless, ignorant. Given the specific circumstances, you can swipe out one adjective and replace it with just about any unflattering descriptor. After a while, the adjectives seem to justify your dislike of the person. You tell yourself, "I don't like him/her. After all, I have seen how *rude* s/he is!!!!!"

Misattribution of meaninglessness is our human folly. We assume that other people's lives are less meaningful. We believe our time is more valuable. We assume their goals are worth less. And we judge our accomplishments as worth more. Our teenagers do it when they ignore our advice in favor of advice from their friends or when they ignore their younger siblings in favor of same-age peers. We do it when we call Mom, Aunt Angie, or Aunt Ida at a moment's notice to baby-sit for us, because—after all—she's retired and bound to be free, right? Professionals do it when they assume people in other professions aren't as important or as knowledgeable. We offer another's credentials as the reason to distrust him/her. "Don't listen to him. After all, he's just a [fill-in the undesirable profession or category here]." We make it a principle to denigrate individuals with whom we disagree, and we give more credence to negative information about them than to positive information (Asch, 1946; Kanouse & Hanson, 1972). "Don't pay attention to her. She's only a ...." We feel justified, vindicated, and elevated when we relegate them to the "trivial" and "not-to-be-trusted" categories. People "discount" other people, and they often do it in order to enhance their own feelings of worth. We convince ourselves that self-worth is a "zero-sum" game, whereby others must be less, so that we can be more (Baumeister, Smart, & Boden, 1996).

How does the consideration of personal worth relate to the creation of eldercare programs and activities? It is the starting point. When we overcome the tendency to devalue others (whether they are children, other adults, individuals with special needs, senior citizens...), then we begin to make contact with the importance of all people and the moments of their lives. When we begin to act as if each human has unquestioned, intrinsic value—regardless of gender, race, ethnic origin, age, background, education, or socioeconomic status—then we can begin to re-value ourselves and others. When we avoid the trap of value-by-comparison, then we can see that there is no benefit in discounting others. We are freed from comparison, and free from diminishing each other, because WE ALL HAVE VALUE SIMPLY BECAUSE WE SHARE THE HUMAN CONDITION. [4] When we let go of our plan to make others less so that we can be more, we not only release them from unfair attributions, we also release ourselves. How so? Not one of us can live up to the person-on-a-pedestal status. Oh, sure! You might be better at volleyball than one friend, or you might be better at math than another, but *sooner or later, you will run into someone who is better than you are at just about everything you think you do best.* And then what will you do?

About Valuing Seniors

For the seniors who are around us—whether they are our spouses, peers, parents, grandparents, or the strangers with whom we come in contact—we can help them to value themselves. We can help them to more fully experience meaning in life when we behave in ways that clearly show that we: 1) value the moments of their lives as just as important as the moments of our lives, and 2) provide support for activities in which they can find meaning. *We succeed when we appreciate the value of other people and help them to spend their moments doing things they find worthwhile!*

In this book, you will find content-oriented chapters that are designed to focus on six areas in the psychology of aging and eldercare. One goal is to help you to foster meaningful experience in the lives of people for whom you provide care. Information is presented around the topics: sensation and movement; perception; thinking and memory; emotion; spirituality and faith; and creativity. Through these six key topics, we can build activities for seniors that: 1) demonstrate to them that they are valuable, and 2) support the elements of self that require routine nurturing, regardless of a person's age.

About Circus Peanuts, the Lawrence Welk Show, and Hats on Cats

The curious reader might wonder about my history and my personal investment in gerontology. Why should anyone listen to what I have to say about eldercare? My affinity for it originated decades ago when, as a preschooler, I regularly visited a "home" with my mom. It was back when eldercare in the USA was in transition from homes [which were actually *houses* where several (often) unrelated elders might live with a nurse or other healthcare professional] to the "long-term care facilities" we have today.[5]

Once every couple weeks, my mom and I would meet her best friend and my best friend (who also happened to be a twenty-something mom and her preschool-aged daughter!). Off we'd go to the "big house with all the nice old people" (a recollection of my three-year-old perception of the event). We'd arrive through the back door of this grand old house as five or six senior citizens were making their way slowly and carefully down the tall oak staircase. The heavy banister supported their weight as they gripped it and stepped with intention. I watched with an eagle eye for the "happy man with those circus peanuts". He was the one who always brought a bag of banana-flavored, bright orange, marshmallow circus peanut candies to share with us. As soon as he had found a seat in the large living room, my best friend and I would lunge toward him. His eyes would sparkle as he inquired, "Do you want a peanut?"

When we had munched a few candies, our mothers would call for us to sit down, and the singing would commence. Hymns, anthems, and favorites: I sang with gusto and verve as I mused, "We sound great!" Now, as I consider that I was only three or four years old and with no ability to read the words in the hymnal, I'm convinced that it was the fun and the smiles that fueled the enjoyment of those involved—and *not* the minstrel quality of our music! As I reminisce about those experiences, I realize how important my parents were in fostering appreciation of the wisdom and wit that grow with age. Wonderful memories of music, fun, and circus peanuts have bolstered my appreciation for elders.

When I was very young, my sister and I had a regular baby-sitter. She was a teenager—responsible, fun, "hip"—but sometimes she wasn't available. On those evenings, when Mom and Dad had a meeting at church or a "work thing", my sister and I went to stay with an elderly couple whose home was warm and cozy. We would sit in over-stuffed recliners and watch Lawrence Welk on their console television. They *loved* Lawrence Welk, and we would watch it too, because we *loved* to spend time with them in their huge, "snuggly" reclining chairs. Sometimes, they would even let us have a glass of *pop* (something rare, due to Mom's worry about all the sugar and caffeine). Today, whenever I see a re-run of Lawrence Welk, I can't help but stop to watch for a few minutes. I reminisce about those evenings when we would croodle into the comfort of our adopted grandparents' big chairs to sip soda and listen to Lawrence! We felt safe; we felt loved.

Many years after singing for circus peanuts and watching Welk, I was an undergraduate in college with an opportunity to work on aging research. Then-graduate-student Tim Snyder and I would trek out to a long-term care complex where he was conducting studies of retrieval strategies in aging memory. At the time, I wasn't sure where my studies would lead me, but my mom was working on a graduate degree in sociology (specializing in gerontology), and her interests had sparked my curiosity. It was only several years afterward, when I was in graduate school, that I began to appreciate the incredible opportunities I had been given: 1) by my parents—who have gifted their children with a very strong sense of the value of life and the human rights of people of all ages; 2) by those with whom I worked when I was an undergraduate; 3) by professors who helped me to learn about neuroscience and cognitive psychology during graduate school; and 4) by the many college students who still come to my classes with curiosity and a willingness to learn about people of all ages and circumstances.

Among other people and events to foster my passion for eldercare is a very unique and special lady. Constance was an independent woman of sophistication and grace. Her life had been full of professional and social engagements, culture and music, but she had never married. In her eighties, Constance (an alias, to protect her identity) suffered a stroke that left her with near fluent (grammatical and flowing) speech but without a connection to the meanings of most words in her memory. She might say, "How are your toes?" When she meant, "How is your family?" As is often true with fluent aphasia (pronounced "u-fay'zhu": a general term for language problems related to neurological dysfunction), Constance continued to enjoy many of the aspects of life. She loved the sunshine and, occasionally, to try her hands at the piano (at which she had been proficient prior to the stroke). She and I had in common several things, including our affection for music, ballet, hats, and kittens. She had traveled abroad, and we shared a great affection for Italy—especially the city of Venice. Despite her problems with identifying things by their correct names, Constance retained an *understanding* of pictures and their concepts. We might look at a book about Italy, and she would exclaim, "Oh, how good! I saw it." In the next sentence, she might try to name the location, "Oh, I love Blonko" [SIC]. Somehow she could not get from her recollection of the place to a correct verbal label for it. [6]

I visited Constance over many months, and I brought her picture books about our shared interests. We sifted through photos of classic ballets and Europe's grand cities. We giggled over photos of cats who paint (see Busch & Silver, 1994) and cats who donned hats (Schenck, 1999). We shared so much fun, and it just didn't seem to matter that she wasn't using the same nouns I was. She would point to a picture of a tabby cat in a bonnet and exclaim, "Look! This man has a flower on!" And it just didn't matter, because I knew what she meant, and she knew what she meant. And the cat *did look silly*, no matter whether we called him a "cat" or a "man".

Constance was in long-term care through one year and into another, but she was frail. As is so often true for physically fragile elders, a new Autumn brought colder weather and susceptibility to pneumonia. During one of my final visits with her, Constance was very ill. Her breathing was labored and she was sad. She wheezed, "Come back when I am...." She stopped because she could not find the word. I responded, "I will come back on a day when you feel *better*." She nodded, and I placed a gift next to her bed: a little plush kitten. She touched it on the head, as if to pet it, and weakly smiled. "Nice," she sighed and closed her eyes to sleep. She died only days after that, and I have missed her. I have reflected about the fun and the laughter. I have remembered our times together—which had little use for nouns—but which had tremendous need for real sharing and heartfelt caring. Our friendship had deep meaning for both of us. It changed my life.

Banana-flavored circus peanuts, Lawrence Welk's musicians, and frill-topped felines are part of my story. I learn every day in eldercare that people who work in caregiving (whether it's nursing, mental health care, or a related field) rarely tell boring tales about how they came to caregiving and why they stayed. I'm certain that the readers of this book have equally interesting stories to share. A great deal of the intrigue and fascination comes from the incredible lives of the elders about whom we care. Through numerous events and the influences of many people, I found fulfilling work in eldercare and gerontology research. I feel a very strong call to promote a perspective that values all humans— *simply because we all share the human condition.* Through this written work, I hope to convey some part of my passion to help care for society's sages. And while it is true that much of my own research and professional experience has focused on dementia care, it is also true that lots of the principles presented in this volume can be applied very broadly across ages and ability-levels.

If your thoughts have turned toward the circumstances of elder life, then this handbook is for you. Whether the concern is about caring for others or about your own adult years, it can help you to explore some key issues in adulthood and aging. Its topics are broad: from emotional life; to spiritual and social well-being; to thinking and memory; to physical tasks; and beyond! **This book is about every person and about the meaning of time in the life of a human.**

2

Sensation and Movement in Elder Life

"I NEVER MET A CHOCOLATE THAT I DIDN'T LIKE."
  –Linda Grayson

Humans are "sensory beings". We accumulate information through taste, touch, smell, vision, and hearing.[1] As infants, we discover the sphere of human existence via "sensorimotor" experiences, and because we are born without fluent language, many aspects of life are first represented in the mind *wordless*. These thoughts are filled with visual images, melodies and sounds, strong tastes, vivid smells, and incredible touches, but not words. Even as a child develops language and as words form thoughts into sentences and propositions, s/he continues to be a "sentient" being. Despite reliance on language—for information gathering, for communicating, and for formulating logical thoughts—all humans are and continue to be sentient throughout their lives.

When I was a newborn, my "Grampy" (our pet name for my maternal grandfather) gave me a special gift. This cowboy on a horse is one of the first presents I ever received, and memories of it are some of my first rich, sensory recollections. You probably know this type of popular baby toy, because they are very much like the "rubber-squeakies" we give our dogs and cats. They are simple, molded plastic or rubber. A small plastic gadget in the bottom of the toy catches the air as the thing is squeezed, and this causes it to make a sound very much like the quack of a duck.

My entrenched memories include the distinct smell of the plastic, the feel of the cowboy's boot against the roof of my mouth, and the look of his funny blue eyes. You might be thinking, "She has lost it. She thinks she has memories of lying in her crib chewing on a baby toy!" Well, not exactly, because this toy was a favorite throughout my preschool years. I carried it with me, kept it in bed with me, and later used it as a stand-in Ken who would marry my Barbie™ doll. Those early experiences of chewing and smelling and seeing and hearing that cowboy toy made it a significant aspect of my infant and toddler years—so much so that I continued to carry it and play with it and...yes...even occasionally chew on it—well into my fourth year. Sensory and motor interactions with an object (or person) of interest: These are the very behaviors that Piaget (1966/1969) referenced when he described sensorimotor development from birth to two years of age. Even though the focus of cognition might change after two years, the foundation of thinking that derives from sensation and movement (and the pleasure or pain one draws from them) continues throughout life.

If physical sensations weren't important, the arts and music, television and radio, eating dessert, drinking coffee, and... even hugging... would have all died out long ago. If "sensing" were inconsequential, we would not buy millions of aspirin tablets and NSAIDs (non-aspirin analgesics, like acetaminophen) each year to ease headaches, muscle aches, and miscellaneous other body pains. We would not lie awake, restless during a windy midnight thunderstorm as the loose shingle thumps and pounds against the roof. I would not be sitting here wolfing down potato chips and wrestling to increase my chip-chomping between bouts of typing! Mmmmm...scrumptious...chips!

An infant's focus is on the five physical senses in an effort to make sense of the world (with the idiom— "making sense"—revealing the story!). If we remember these lessons of our own development, then we can appreciate the importance of the senses as they continue to make life meaningful—even after infancy. The senses bring us information and they amplify our experiences. We appreciate beauty more when we have sensory experiences directly related to beauty, e.g., seeing an exquisite sunset, watching a fly-ball as it pops up over the stadium crowd, hearing the roar of an ocean wave as it approaches the beach. Notice that sensing can be a very active process. We crave experiences, and we act on the world in order to make more new experiences—when we *turn on* the car radio, *snuggle* under a warm blanket, *switch on* the television, *jog* across a dew-soaked meadow at sunrise, or *churn* homemade ice cream. The resulting sensations (like savoring that sundae!) cause a surge of chemicals (neurotransmitters, such as serotonin and dopamine) in the brain. Those neurotransmitters are linked to feelings of pleasure and the motivation to seek it. Thus, when we are rewarded—through brain chemistry—for seeking music, warmth, sit-com humor, physical exercise, and sugary treats, it increases the chance that we'll seek those sensations again. We experience pleasure, and then we *actively seek* more pleasure (see the classic studies of kittens who actively sought rewards by solving the puzzle of a trap door which stood between them and food; Thorndike, 1898).[2]

Piaget's (1966/1969) term, "sensorimotor", illuminates the role of a human as active when s/he takes in new information about the world. Gibson (1966) called humans "actor-observers" and he contended that 'perception implies action'. That is, we look, we touch, we listen...rather than merely seeing, feeling, hearing....[3]

Even for individuals with physical conditions that limit their activity, cravings for sensory stimulation are alive. There is a vast literature on stimulation-seeking among children of neglect and among individuals in situations of sensory-deprivation (like seeking stimulation by rocking oneself, humming, pacing, or arranging objects in rows; see American Psychiatric Association, 1994). [4] For individuals in long-term care, the attentive touch of a nurse, a nurse's aid, or another caregiver can provide much needed sensory stimulation (Brownlee & Dattilo, 2002). The benefits of touch for elders have been demonstrated even beyond the boundaries of long-term care facilities in the so-called "naturally occurring retirement communities" (often called NORC's; Chow, 2002; Kunstler, 2002). Research on physical touch indicates that it can actually improve immune system function, perceptions of pain, and levels of anxiety (see Hall, Thorns, & Oliver, 2003).

Like many other professionals who work with seniors, I find that one of the most important actions I can take to provide caring through touch is to simply reach out and take another's hand(s) into my hands and to gently hold on with a light caress. If I reach out, as I speak a person's name and make eye contact, then I help the individual to orient and focus and I demonstrate that

I am focused on him/her. This makes a strong statement about my sense of his/her personal worth.

About the Aging Senses: Sight

When we appreciate the role sensations play in our daily lives, we begin to understand their continued importance for adults. Further consider that for older adults time, biology, and circumstances (like exposure to toxins or to harmful stimuli in settings such as industry or one's workplace) might play tricks to alter the senses and to cheat them of sharpness.[5] Even though there are broad individual differences, there are some specific changes in sense organs and systems that do appear commonly in human aging. For example, no matter the visual acuity in childhood and younger adulthood, the average person's elder eyes tend to be more presbyopic (the far-sightedness of advancing age; Kolb & Whishaw, 2006). It is the result of thickening of the optic lens which leads it to be less flexible and, therefore, less able to accommodate (or bend) to focus on proximal (i.e., close) objects (e.g., Kolb & Whishaw; Bee & Boyd, 2002). Thankfully, large print versions of popular books and magazines are available for readers who find it difficult to see standard-sized fonts. For people with low vision, some books are reproduced as audio recordings. If you care for someone who has difficulty reading as a result of poor visual acuity, it might be worthwhile to check with local organizations that offer volunteer services. If a publisher doesn't provide an audio recording of a book, then a volunteer group might be willing to provide you with: 1) reading services for individuals who would like to *hear* a book, magazine, or newspaper, or 2) audio recordings of portions of printed materials (with mindfulness that recording an entire book on tape might require permission from the book's publisher).

With age, and especially after age 60, the eyes are less able to focus on near objects, are less able to register incoming light (because of a thickening lens), and are less able to accurately identify hues (especially the blueness of objects). Also, because the optic lens "yellows" with age and becomes more likely to absorb blue and blue-violet wavelengths of light, it prompts some objects to look more yellow (e.g., Arking, 1991).

In my own research on the arts, I find that elderly participants (e.g., over 70 years) often report a plain white piece of paper to be "yellow". An interesting point can be made about this, as it relates to the "aesthetic quality" of what is seen. The yellowed lens can lead one to see the world as more yellow, and because yellow seems to be humans' *least* preferred color, it might lead to a diminishment of aesthetic experiences and pleasure associated with looking (about color preference, see

McManus, Jones, & Cottrell, 1981). [6] In plain words, some people don't like yellow too much. If they have to look at a *world-turned-yellow*, they might feel *blue!* [7]

The yellowing effect of an aging optic lens can often be counteracted with lights and visual stimuli that tend toward the blue-violet end of the visible spectrum (i.e., below about 500 mµ). It is unfortunate that so many contemporary architects and builders are infatuated with "rose" and "orange" hued fluorescent lights (e.g., above 600 mµ). Although they save electricity (and are, therefore, very cost-effective), this choice in lighting is often hapless for elders, who might experience glare and yellowing made worse by fluorescent lights and their aging vision (—not to mention the few residents and staff whose migraines or seizures can be triggered by the flicker of fluorescent lights and some TV/computer displays; see Harding & Jeavons, 1994). [8] These rose and orange lights, if chosen for aesthetic reasons, have most likely been selected as a result of misunderstanding the complicated literature on color, lighting, and aesthetic preference (Davidoff, 1991; see his Ch. 8).

About counteracting the yellowing effect of an aging eye, an example can elucidate. Without mentioning my purpose, I handed a stack of "baby blue" art paper to a 92-year-old participant in one of my activity groups. She is high-functioning, active, and is often a leader in group activities. After a few minutes during which I had yet to explain the stack of paper to her, she looked at it and asked, "What should I do with this white paper, Honey?" The pale blueness of the paper was probably counteracted by the yellowing of her vision and the very bright, "orange" fluorescent lights of the activity room. The result was her perception of the paper as white.

About the Aging Senses: Sound

If vision is the sense we depend on most, then a close second is hearing. We rely on it to help us speak and to help us understand what is said. However, audition does change with age. Overall, hearing at higher frequencies (from 2,000 Hz and up) diminishes with age—especially beyond age 70 (see Arking, 1991, p. 178; Whitbourne, 1985). This phenomenon is called presbycusis, and it appears in increasing numbers of people after age thirty (along with mild loss of very low frequencies during midlife; Kirasic, 2004; Arking, 1991). In a report about incidence of hearing problems in middle adulthood that was based on National Health Interview Survey statistics, Adams and Benson (1992; Kirasic, p. 65) noted that 179 males and 107 females out of every 1,000 mid-lifers had some hearing difficulty. For middle-aged and older adults, speech (particularly of higher pitched voices like those of women and children) can become more difficult to discern. Thus, considerations about one's speaking volume are critical—especially for those of us whose voices are of higher pitch (Bee & Boyd, 2002).

Activities for elders that are directed by a person with a high-pitched voice or designed around high-frequency sounds must accommodate presbycusis by increasing volume (without using a higher pitch). It is preferable for presented sounds to include a range, with emphases on mid- and lower-range pitches (below 2,000 Hz when possible). Sound emphasis on high frequencies (2,000 Hz or above; Kirasic, 2004, p. 66) is a mistake in eldercare, especially when conditions are noisy, because sounds can "mask" each other, and high frequencies are more susceptible to be camouflaged in noisy environments (see Blumenfeld, Bergman, & Millner, 1969; Bergman, 1971). In a classic paper on speech discrimination among adults, Bergman et al. (1976) demonstrated that beyond age 30, individuals showed impairments understanding human speech. The most marked problems were among those aged over 50 years and among the most degraded speech conditions (such as echoing speech that might occur in a large room and "crackling", broken speech that one might hear on a telephone or cellular phone). Tun (1998) reported evidence that group differences between younger and older adults in speech discernment are "magnified" by a noisy environment and by speeded speech. Overall, it seems very likely that problems discerning high frequencies—especially high-pitched speech—contribute to an overall advantage of younger over older adult hearing (as in the cross-sectional effect reported by Bergman et al.; also, as discussed by Schaie & Willis, 2002).

When I speak to elders in an activity group, I try to look directly at them, using very few head movements for the duration of my utterance (because head movements can be distracting and can disrupt lip-reading). I speak in the lower pitch register of my voice, and more loudly than usual, so that they have the best opportunity to hear me. I also enunciate slightly more slowly, because speech recognition can be more impaired when speaking rates are faster (Bergman et al., 1976; Gordon-Salant & Fitzgibbons, 1999). Specifically, for individuals with dementia, eye contact is especially important, because it helps them to focus on the speaker. I often begin by stating the listener's name very clearly as I look directly at him/her. This helps to orient the individual to listen (see Dowling, 1995; Mace, 1989; Bell & Troxel, 1997, pp. 116-117). Eye contact also demonstrates aspects of caring: 1) commitment to attend to another person, and 2) willingness to invest time in conversation with him/her. Notice, too, that "conversation" can include many ways of communicating—such as non-verbal gestures, facial expressions, and non-linguistic vocalizations. An individual with moderate-to-severe dementia might still be able to communicate using non-verbal gestures (Baker, 2005), and a person who has experienced language disruption because of a left, frontal lobe stroke might yet be able to communicate, even if his/her speech is not fluent (Sife, 1998).

About the Aging Senses: Scents

In *Remembrance of Things Past*, Proust (1927) reminisced about the significance of smell and the other senses as cues to memory. Unfortunately, because the sense of smell deteriorates in late life, activities that focus on smell are not a good choice for senior citizens. This is especially true for individuals with probable Alzheimer's disease, in which olfactory deficits are pronounced (see Vance, 2002). Because noticing and identifying specific odors declines significantly after age 60, activities that utilize smell should include additional cues from other senses (such as the sight of a pretty flower or the sounds of seagulls and waves). The other senses can provide a focus for senior activities which smell cannot (Doty, Reyes, & Gregor, 1987).

Application: How the Senses Cue Memory to Stimulate Action

In a sensory-cognitive activity that I have used often among groups with moderate Alzheimer's disease (AD), I distribute silk flowers of many different varieties. [9] Each participant (with ladies usually preferring this task) has three or four flowers in front of her on the table. I begin by telling them that we'll be discussing flowers and gardening today. I continue, "I'm going to call out a particular type of flower. If you have that one, then hold it up!" The game consists of rounds, and during each one, just one type of flower is called. For example: "I'm calling all sunflowers. Please, pass in your sunflower."

For every type of flower I call, I can circulate around the table and ask each participant to add one of hers to an arrangement of that flower type (which I've already started making in a sturdy plastic vase). I announce, "Whoever gets rid of her flowers first will win the game!" When the "game" is up, we have several beautiful arrangements. [*Without* the goal of making an arrangement to spur them on, many participants with Alzheimer-type dementia (DAT; i.e., cognitive impairment associated with Alzheimer's disease) will prefer to keep their flowers. The arrangements make nice individual prizes or decorations for a "commons" area—where everyone can enjoy them. If you don't set up a goal (like making flower arrangements), that's okay. However, you should be prepared for an argument when you try to get all your flowers back!]

It is striking to me that participants in the "flower game" hold the silk flowers up to their noses repeatedly and sniff them—as if these buds and blossoms were freshly cut. They say, "Mmmm," or "Ahhh!"— seemingly unaware that the blooms smell like silk and plastic. One group member might lean over to another and beseech her, "Honey, smell this one! Isn't it gorgeous?" This is an excellent example of powerful visual information that can prompt one to smell or sniff—even when the nose cannot discern the difference between a floral-scented bloom and an unscented silk flower. What is critical is that the visual cues lead one into an automatized or "procedural" memory for enjoying flowers which includes gazing at them, holding them by the stem, sniffing them, and reacting with verbal exclamations of glee! Presumably, flower gazing and blossom sniffing have been practiced a lot in many people's lives.

Given the deterioration of many elders' sense of smell, it is highly unlikely that olfactory cues could lead the flower game in the same way that visual aspects commandeer it (Vance, 2002). Cueing procedural memories (like memories for highly practiced sequences such as folding laundry or assembling a specific puzzle; Poe & Seifert, 1997) is one of the most useful techniques in activity programming for individuals with Alzheimer's disease and related dementias, because memories for highly practiced activities can persist even as memories for facts and events decline (Knopman & Nissen, 1987). In one study, Mindy (Poe) Baker and I observed that elderly individuals got faster at assembling a wooden puzzle—even when they could not recall having assembled it previously (Poe & Seifert). [10]

Application: It's Natural to
Build Fun around Food

Taste is related to smell, chemically (e.g., Pinel, 2003). Diminished smell can reduce the intensity of taste. If we add to that the routine loss of taste buds and a decrease in saliva production with age (which can be even more profound, depending on one's eating, smoking, and health habits; but see Bornstein & Lamb, 1999) ,[11] then taste's decline is clearly another issue in aging. However, taste remains a critical part of life across the life-span—both because *eating is intrinsically pleasurable* and because *eating is a social activity* (not to mention eating in order to stay alive). In the very early years of my research on dementia care, I was having some difficulty finding volunteers for a memory study. One of my mentors suggested that I make cookies. She put it this way, "If you bring food, then it's an event!" Since then, I have had no problem gathering volunteers for my research studies—as long as I bring goodies! Moreover, with the recent advances in sugar substitutes, there are abundant products available so that individuals with diabetes can participate, too. Thus, taste continues to be important for seniors, and the diminished intensity of flavors requires us to take more care to consider other aspects of gastronomy: like food texture, temperature, and appearance. One of the favorite snacks for participants in my Tuesday-Thursday evening "Reflections" group (for individuals with memory decline) was strawberry ice cream. It's cool; it's sweet; and it's bright pink!

As it relates to food and fun, an undergraduate student once scolded me with, "Dr. Seifert, you've always taught us that we shouldn't use food as a reward, because food is very emotional. What about all those lectures when you've said we shouldn't train our children to do things by rewarding with candy, dessert, or soda pop?" My response: a general rule that excludes food rewards can be very healthy for children. Then, they won't be as likely to seek out food as solace or as prone to eat in order to squelch firestorms of emotion. Conversely, for someone who has reached the eighth or ninth decade of life, a delicious snack can be just the ticket to encourage eating and socializing![12] This sentiment was expressed to me bluntly by a gentleman in one of my activity groups when he grinned and hollered, "I see candy; gimme, gimme, gimme. I'm an old man and haven't got time to wait!" In response to his remark, the entire group burst into laughter!

 Application: About the Power of Touch

With respect to touch, the related somatosensations are a person's impressions about what's happening to his/her body, like a feeling of pain, a sense of one's own body movement, and a sense of one's self in three-dimensional space. These abilities to monitor one's body can shift with age, but the ways they change are multifaceted. Some sensations like light touch (as in sensing a feather that brushes across the skin) and deep touch (like the feeling of pressure when someone in a crowd bumps into you) deteriorate little with age—despite some anatomical alterations in their primary receptors (Arking, 1991). It seems that only the face and hands (which are exposed more often to light and weather than other areas of the body) experience a significant decrease in sensitivity to touch over time. Other aging changes in sensations of body position, movement, and pain seem to be highly individualized, even though some aspects of pain and temperature discernment might be dulled, overall (Bornstein & Lamb, 1999). One moderating factor for all aging individuals is change in musculo-skeletal integrity (Kirasic, 2004). The natural "suspension system" for joints, muscles, and bones deteriorates from midlife on, and this makes us less bendable and more prone to movement-associated injuries. Also, muscle mass declines with aging, decreasing one's overall strength. Indeed, the strength of one's grip generally drops from age 29 and after (Kirasic).

When I teach classes about eldercare, I suggest the shoulders as an excellent location for a caring touch from a caregiver's or nurse aid's/assistant's hand, because the shoulders experience little change in touch sensation with age. Moreover, a shoulder can be a "safe spot", which is not usually associated with sexual advances (per Title IX and the Civil Rights Acts of 1964; consult the U.S. EEOC, 2003). The issue about intimate advances (or perceived advances) should not be ignored, because research on sexuality reveals that elders are not the "asexual" beings whom younger cohorts would suppose them to be (Tan, 2005; Marshall, 2006; Bitzer & Alder, 2003; Whitbourne, 2001, Meston, 1997; DiGiovanna, 1994; Vonsydow, 1992; Ludeman, 1981). Thus, as is generally true of interpersonal interactions between caregiver and care-receiver (except perhaps in relationships like a person caring for his/her spouse), efforts should be made NOT to communicate a sexual message (U.S. EEOC). A nurse's aid might protest, "How can I draw these boundaries for residents when I'm charged with *bathing* residents and helping them use the *toilet*?" One key is to draw the distinction between the specific event of bathing (or toileting) and other events that involve touch. A common technique is to train nurse's aids to utilize specific behaviors, directions, and/or voice tones during bath and toilet tasks that are not used during casual social interactions (such as those related to food, games, and chit-chat). Another method is to divide tasks between aids, so that there are specific aids who administer baths and assist toileting and others who do not. [This is an admittedly more difficult method—being somewhat less desirable for those aids who are assigned to bath and toilet duties.] Despite complex issues about privacy and sexuality, overall, touch remains a critical part of personal care, and I'll discuss more about that issue in the application section below (see also, Hartz & Splain, 1997).

Application: About the Five Senses in Eldercare

When we design activities for eldercare, particularly for individuals who have cognitive decline (e.g., due to stroke, vascular dementia, Alzheimer's disease), sensory stimuli can play a principal part. For individuals who have normal cognitive function, multimodal (i.e., stimulating more than one sense) experiences can be wonderful. 1) Eating popcorn while watching a movie that contains favorite melodies from one's youth; 2) listening to a musical performer while enjoying an opportunity to dance or sing along (if one is physically able); 3) participating in a special event with foods, sports-spectating, songs, and/or costumes (like a luau, a sock-hop, or a St. Patrick's Day party); 4) taking part in preparations for an upcoming holiday or celebration by making craft items and listening to thematic music; or 5) any number of other events that involve more than one of the senses: These are all excellent activities for eldercare—especially when individuals are normal functioning or have only mild cognitive impairments.

Multi-modal events can, however, be overwhelming for persons with dementia, cognitive decline, and related conditions. We must be careful to consider 1) the current state of one's sensory systems, and 2) one's cognitive abilities. If an individual has probable Alzheimer's disease ("pAD": a diagnosis made from behavioral and cognitive symptoms when a definitive physiological or genetic marker for AD isn't available) and has progressed beyond very mild cognitive impairment, then s/he might be highly distractible. Multi-modal inputs (like a party in a brightly lighted room with lots of conversation and music) could produce "sensory overload". S/he might not be able to focus on any single detail of the incoming "stimuli" (another word for "pieces of information"). S/he might become confused and act on that confusion by hitting, yelling, falling due to disorientation in space, or worse. One point that is made in many books and articles on dementia care is that we can improve the quality of an experience by reducing distractions (e.g., Zgola, 1987; Sheridan, 1987; Bell & Troxel, 1997).

One of my former students, Chris Szostak (Szostak & Seifert, 2001), designed a multi-modal activity for individuals with mild-to-moderate Alzheimer-type dementia. We played audiotaped versions of common sounds while participants viewed black line drawings (of about 2 in X 4 in; i.e., 5.08 cm X 10.16 cm) mounted on 5 in X 7 in (12.70 cm X 17.78 cm) white index cards. In front of each participant, we placed several of these cards with drawings on them (i.e., one corresponding drawing and several "incorrect" drawings; with the latter type of drawings also being called "foils" or "distracters"). One goal of the task was for participants to listen to a sound (like a train engine with a whistle, the buzz of a bumble-bee, or a ringing school bell) and then point to the corresponding picture (a train engine, a bee, or a school bell). Unfortunately, participants with probable Alzheimer's disease seemed to have great difficulty integrating sights (i.e., the line drawing) with sounds (emitted by a cassette recorder). We were fairly sure that the problem was not sound detection, because participants would look toward the source of the sound and ask, "What is that?" or "Why don't you shut that off?" Thus, they were *hearing* the sounds. Apparently, though, the simple line drawings were not salient (i.e., noticeable) enough and were too far removed from the sounds to be perceived as related to them. When we eliminated the pictures and presented sounds alone, participants seemed somewhat more likely to identify (by naming) the sounds and their sources [— although they did still experience some difficulties— which we attribute, in part, to the noxious aspect of a few of the sounds (as startling and unpleasant; e.g., the buzzing bee)]. It seems as if the sounds required all of their attention, so that none was left over for looking at the pictures!

When I reflect on the failure of integration across pictures and sound effects in Chris Szostak's (Szostak & Seifert, 2001) pilot study, I recall two similar phenomena: one that Davidoff and Mitchell (1993) observed in pre-school aged children, and another that I observed among young adults (Seifert, 1997). Davidoff and Mitchell reported a color recognition activity in which they had asked children under 5 years of age to identify the real-world colors of common objects and animals. Some children responded to a verbal query such as "What is the right color of a horse? Brown or green?" and some responded to pictures, "Here are two pictures of a horse. Which is the right color, that one or that one?" (pointing to pictures; with my examples synthesized from their list of stimuli and description of procedures; see their p. 125 and Appendix 1). They reported that the children had great difficulty selecting the correct line drawing when an inappropriately colored drawing was also in the field of view. Davidoff and Mitchell reported that children had much less difficulty with an object-color identification when they viewed an uncolored drawing (presumably black lines on white paper; see Snodgrass & Vanderwart, 1980) or were asked to name the correct real-world color (their Study 2). Davidoff and Mitchell's results indicate that the miscolored pictures were pulling the young children's attention away from the correct responses, and pictures appeared to do this in a way that verbal probes did not.

In a completely different study, I observed similar effects of distraction by picture "foils" (i.e., unrelated pictures). In this experiment young adults had been asked to look at pairs of items (some picture pairs and some word pairs) on a computer screen (Seifert, 1997). I asked the participants to press buttons to respond "yes" or "no" to the query: "Are the two items related in any way?" It seemed to me that subjects were experiencing hesitations on "no" responses to picture pairs. Several participants must have thought this as well, because they offered unsolicited excuses for the response delay on unrelated picture pairs. They claimed to be slowed down by imagining associations between the two things—merely as a result of seeing the two items pictured together. My guess is that the unrelated items, pictured together, distracted the participants to think about ways in which the two items *could be associated* (especially by using visual imagery to think about the objects and how they might interact in physical space). This did not seem to happen when they viewed pairs of words.

A common issue across Chris Szostak's (Szostak & Seifert, 2001) sound study, Davidoff and Mitchell's (1993) color study, and my (Seifert, 1997) association-recognition task is: that it is very possible to (presumably unwittingly) build distractions into an activity, and some stimuli will be more distracting than others. *As a general rule, it is the nature of the participants that will help you to determine whether they are able to recover from the distraction.* In my memory studies of young adults, the distraction from unrelated picture pairs robbed them of mere fractions of a second, and they were able to bring themselves back to the task quickly to respond "no" (i.e., that the items were not related). In Davidoff and Mitchell's study, many children seemed unable to recover from visual distraction by an inappropriately colored drawing. Their average score was 77.74% correct in *selecting the spoken name* of an object's usual color versus 55.97% correct in *pointing to a correctly colored drawing* while also looking at wrong-colored foils (see their pp. 126-127; with performance being as much as 21.77% diminished because of visual distraction)! Similarly, in Chris Szostak's sound activity, participants with Alzheimer's disease seemed unable to recover from startle responses to sounds. With their attention pulled away by a sound, they seemed unable to recover quickly enough to look at pictures of objects that might make such a sound. By the time their attention had been redirected to the line drawings, the sound was forgotten (i.e., probably due to the impairment in short-term memory which accompanies AD). [13]

How can we design activities that integrate two or more senses? Contrast the aforementioned failure to integrate across sense modalities (in Szostak's sound study; Szostak & Seifert, 2001) with the success we see in a game of charades. In our version of charades, an activity leader acts out examples from a specified category (e.g., animals, actions, or musical instruments; an activity which Mindy Baker helped to develop; see Seifert, 1999). I might get down "on all fours" and say, "Mooooo!" [Oh, yes! This game is fun, and participants have a great laugh. They love to tease the one who acts out the charades!] I think that this task owes its success to its ability to keep participants focused on the source of the sound (i.e., the group leader), despite the fact that the leader doesn't *look* like a cow (or a violin, or a vacuum cleaner). Because s/he is in the center of the group and everyone is attending to the charade gestures, it is almost automatic for participants to yell out the correct response once they see an integrated set of gestures and sounds. Again, notice that the sounds and gestures occur together and *in the same location in space*. Thus, charades don't present the same problem of integrating sense modalities across space and time that Chris Szostak and I observed in our sounds and pictures study (which was described above). [14]

For individuals with Alzheimer's disease and related types of dementia, one key to utilizing multiple sense modalities is to help maintain attention *without* precipitating sensory overload. Generally, persons with normal cognitive function (or with mild dementia) will be able to tolerate more sensory stimulation than individuals with moderate-to-severe cognitive impairments. In my experience supervising activities, I've gathered that people with moderate AD can handle about 30-40 minutes of charades before they need to "cool down" with a snack or a quiet activity.

I orient the group with moderate AD to a game of charades by leading 8 to 15 of them into a well-lighted (preferably with natural light) activity room (of approximately 25 ft X 25 ft). We set up for the game in an "auditorium style" gathering—with the activity leader standing at the front of the room and with participants seated in a semicircular arrangement around the leader. This facilitates communication, because the leader is near enough to any given individual to be heard and to hear possible responses as participants call them out. It also helps the leader to keep participants' attention, because they are close enough to make casual conversation with them in-between individual charades (see Seifert, 1999, for a study of specific charades and research results).

In charades, if I act out a "cow", and hear the correct response, I can proceed to make a joke that will fuel conversation. To the individual who guesses, "Cow," I might grin and respond, "[Participant's name here], did you just call me a cow? Oh, dear! What will I tell my husband? I'll have to tell him, 'Honey, you married a cow. Moooooo!' And what do you think he'll say to that?" All this conversation is part of the art of making simple activities more age-appropriate for adults with cognitive impairments. And we *must* know our audience members, too. There are some folks who would respond to my joking with wit of their own, but there are others who might misunderstand it as childish, or worse, as mockery *of them*. These are the folks who shake their heads and wander out of the room with a disapproving frown. It's critical to gauge respondents and their potential reactions to you.[15] One key to a successful activity is to include those who are most likely to enjoy the activity (based on accurate information about an individual's history, preferences, and current behaviors). Don't try to entice or coerce participation—especially by those who are likely to be bored, annoyed, or deeply frustrated by the experience.

If I want to interest a shy, demure participant who has guessed, "Cow," then I might respond by looking down and saying, "Oh, and don't I look silly. Why don't I try something a bit more challenging like everyday actions? This next one is an activity that we adults engage in before we leave the house in the morning." Now, I have acknowledged the silliness of the animal category and I can engage the more sophisticated observer by acting out "putting on a coat", "brushing teeth", or an even more select activity like "a man putting on a neck tie" or "a woman putting on lipstick" (Seifert, 1999; with some of these examples added to the task after the 1999-article was published). It's all part of trying to engage participants in activities that affirm them. One critical element is to know which residents/clients are the best candidates for particular activities or projects. Individuals who love to play games, who like to compete, and who have high needs for affiliation with other people are usually better candidates for games like charades than are those who are more quiet, shy, and introverted. The latter individuals might be better candidates for one-on-one conversations, reading groups, "lecture" formats, and "table activities" (see Sheridan, 1987; Zgola, 1987; Dowling, 1995; Bell & Troxel, 1997).

Application: Individualized Needs for Affiliation and Involvement

As Zgola (1987, p. 35) has discussed, at the highest level of participation, individuals can plan, organize, and conduct an event like a party, dance, or creative project. That is what normal functioning adults do—whether they are 29 or 79. They find meaning in creating events in life. Building meaning is a fundamental process of human existence. [16]

However, as Zgola (1987) and others have observed, cognitive and health declines can interfere with one's ability to plan, organize, and bring to fruition a meaningful activity. Here are opportunities for a caregiver, an aid, or an activities professional to provide help. If a person has Parkinson's disease (which impairs motor movements and their execution), I might engage him/her in the aspects of planning an event. However, I might delegate a lot of the physical labor (like blowing up and tying balloons or filling small party bags with candy/prizes) to someone else who is more able to carry out tasks of fine coordination. [17] If an individual is in the early stages of probable Alzheimer's disease (and without physical impairments), I might include him/her in all aspects of planning and execution of an event. However, I would be present at all stages, in order to keep him/her "on task", because short-term memory problems might prompt someone to wander from his/her plan (for examples of structured memory support of this type see Seifert, 2000; also, Zgola, 1990).[18]

In an article from the millennium year, I described an individualized project for a lady with mild dementia of the Alzheimer-type (Seifert, 2000). She cherished a family heirloom, and it had begun to deteriorate from age. In consultation with her and with her family, I designed a set of activities to assist as she refurbished the heirloom. The steps in the task were fitted to her affinity for handiwork, and they were tailored to her needs for frequent reminders (a result of her difficulties with short-term memory). I fit the reminders into conversation as she and I worked together to bring the heirloom back to some of its former beauty. Overall, my knowledge of this lady's history, specific cognitive problems, and personal preferences were key as I helped her to act on her world in a meaningful and fulfilling way (Seifert).

My 2000-article about customized activities is consistent with one of the most useful methods of caring for people with special needs (whether they are 2 or 102 years old): with "person-centered" care being an incredibly valuable approach (Cotrell & Schulz, 1993; Kitwood, 1993; see also Bell & Troxel, 1997; Woods, 2001; Barnes et al., 2002). In nursing care, a person-centered approach—which also regards one's culture, the culture of care, and the universal aspects of compassion—has been described by Leininger and McFarland (2006). A main idea of both approaches (i.e., Kitwood's person-centered approach to eldercare and Leininger and McFarland's theory of cultural care in nursing) is that person care requires real, customized "caring" for an individual who receives care.

Greenspan and Wieder (1998) described person-centered care for children with special needs in terms of a tiered prioritization scheme. Their prescription for individualized care can be applied to eldercare, and the approach seems to derive loosely from Maslow's hierarchy of human needs (e.g., Maslow, 1970). According to Maslow, the most essential human needs are "physiological". They are, for example, the requirements of the body for sustenance and nutrition. Second to those are "safety" needs—like having a sense of predictability in one's life. People also have needs for love, attention, and affiliation with others. Beyond those needs, we must feel competent and worthwhile (called "esteem" needs). Ultimately, Maslow believed that we all have a need to reach for our individual potential—at the pinnacle of human aspirations—which he called the ongoing process of "self-actualizing".

It has been argued that Abraham Maslow later added a sixth level of need to his hierarchy, which involves transcendence of self (Maslow, 1970; see Koltko-Rivera, 2006). Personally, I believe that true self-actualizing must involve a process of optimizing self *through transcendence.* Therefore, my adapted hierarchy for eldercare interventions (Table 1, below; Appendix A, this book) incorporates the possibility for experiences of peak value that are beyond the self and which might involve communion with others (and, even, the universe).

Maslow (1970) described lower needs in the hierarchy as "prepotent", i.e., generally usurping higher needs. If I'm severely famished, then presumably I'll search for food, rather than lounge about and contemplate the meaning of "social justice". Here's the caveat to that rule: that once an individual has experienced the liberating influence of higher needs, s/he might very well sacrifice satisfaction at lower levels of the hierarchy for fulfillment at higher levels. Consider a monk who fasts for days or weeks in order to de-focus from bodily cravings in favor of reflection about life's meaning. One of Maslow's points was that so-called "peak experiences"—which occur when one seeks to live up to his/her potential—can displace lower-level needs from priority. Even if the monastic is starving, s/he might forego food in favor of the peak experience of breaking through to understand life's essence. That type of behavior is not reserved for people in cloisters and monasteries; millions of members of organized religions routinely fast in order to focus on prayer, supplication, and worship.

Two books about integrated care relate intervention approaches that incorporate Maslow's (1970) hierarchy of needs. Greenspan and Wieder's (1998) model of "integrated... intervention" for children with special needs begins with "[b]asic services for safety, security, and protection" (p. 379; after Maslow). In a similar turn, Bowlby (1993) described an application of Maslow's needs to dementia care. In her approach, Bowlby explained that individuals with AD and related disorders can still achieve even the highest level of need fulfillment (i.e., self-actualizing). Perhaps the major difference between persons with dementia and people without dementia is the level of environmental/social support (e.g., from caregivers, family, nursing home staff) necessary to assist in achieving satisfied need states (especially, Bowlby, pp. 80-83 and Ch. 5). I have adapted ideas from both books to create a set of steps for 'integrated interventions' in eldercare (in Table 1).

Table 1: Infusing Interventions into Individualized Care*

Step 1: Ensuring nutrition, physical well-being, and basic care of a person with special needs (combining Maslow's two foundational levels of need: health and safety);

Step 2: Providing support for integrity in relationships (per Maslow's needs for love and belonging);

Step 3: Arranging interactions which are aimed at one's personal abilities and the needs for sensing stimuli, interpreting incoming information, and planning actions (per Maslow's esteem needs);

Step 4: Utilizing intervention strategies that *foster development*; Also, for elders, *promoting independence* (when possible) and supporting one's current level of functioning (per Maslow's esteem needs and toward self-actualization); and

Step 5: Enacting person-centered interventions motivated by specific history, preferences, personality, and the potential of the individual who receives care (per Maslow's concept of self-actualization); And using personal history to transform optimal functioning *in context* when/if possible

* Ideally, all steps occur together in an integrated care plan. My list is expanded beyond, but adapted from Greenspan and Wieder's (1998, Ch. 18, p. 379; also, see Appendix A of this volume). I use the term "special needs" to refer to persons who might require assistance from others in goal-seeking and in satisfying needs.

Consider the importance of individual differences in the ways elders interact with their world (about individual differences in personality change see, Warner et al., 2004). An example is the case of a gentleman older than ninety, living in a long-term care facility. He had emigrated from China and was isolated, in many ways, from the USA-born residents of the facility because of: 1) his accent (i.e., when speaking English), 2) the unwillingness of other residents/peers to try to understand his speech, and 3) his desire for more frequent visits from family (admittedly a common want among elders, whose adult children might be attentive but still busy raising their own families and attending to their careers and homes). This gentleman—shy and humble—required merely a quiet conversation of 10 – 15 minutes daily with a specified staff member in order to improve in mood, in motivation to eat and exercise, and in his willingness to trust facility staff. His needs for excitement, for noise, for visual stimulation (with his vision being poor) were very modest. But his need for a confidant—for someone he knew as *his* pal—was high. This example illustrates the essence of integrated, person-centered care. His physiological and safety needs were met by the facility's medical/nursing staff. His needs to trust others at the facility, to maintain command of spoken English, to be engaged socially in conversation, and to have specific conversations about individual interests (levels 2 through 5 above, respectively) were met by activities staff and volunteers. Without conversation and social interaction (to satisfy needs 2 through 5), meeting his physiological needs (e.g., for food and water) seemed to bring him little satisfaction.

An application of Maslow's (1970) need hierarchy to eldercare would be incomplete without considering Bennett's (1980) innovative research. Bennett entered long-term care as a participant-observer and played the role of man with a history of alcohol abuse. He reported his experience as "very incarcerating", and he disliked being "lumped together" with others who had many, varied medical troubles and cognitive impairments (Bennett, p. 59). In addition, Bennett surveyed residents in long-term care to discern their greatest self-reported sense of need. The unexpected outcome was that one's possessions were listed foremost as a need. Bennett (and later Hartz & Splain, 1997) pointed to the loss of possessions which typically occurs when one moves into long-term care (or into an apartment, a group home, or the home of one's adult child). This can precipitate a sense of great loss. I add the following point to their interpretations: **that the possessions people collect during their lives are** *symbols* **of accomplishments, feats, and triumphs. By extension** *possessions symbolize who the person is.*

I have a friend who played football in high school. It has been a long time since he was fit enough to compete with seventeen-year-olds, yet he once did. His football memorabilia remind him of those days—of a time when he was competitive—and he derives a sense of meaning from those. He plans to give some of those mementos to his children. In a way, this bequest represents a gift of part of himself to them. The mementos represent an aspect of the meaning of his life and a way in which he'd like to be remembered.

Not only for someone with normal cognitive function, but for an individual with dementia, possessions can serve as needed cues to otherwise dimming memories about his/her identity and accomplishments. It is beyond me to count the elders with whom I've worked over the years who have had probable Alzheimer's disease and who have exhibited repetitive searching and hiding behaviors. One case comes to mind of a woman with a relatively severe impairment of short-term memory and a moderate deficit in long-term memory. She would spend hours searching for a treasured photo. Upon finding it, she would exclaim, "There he is! There is *my heart*," about this just-recovered photo of her husband. Immediately, she would set about to find a "special place" to hide the photo for "safe-keeping". Then, often within minutes, she would be panic-stricken again that the picture was "gone" or "lost" (or worse still, "stolen"). The advent of inexpensive photo-imaging and copying technologies has been a God-send, because we can stock-pile copies of these precious photos and bring them out when the original has been temporarily misplaced. Some families prefer to store original photos for safekeeping and make some color copies of them available to a loved one with dementia. Inexpensive copies can be handled (and sometimes hidden) by a person with dementia, without sending everyone into panic mode when they are tattered or lost.

In cases like the one I've just described, it is folly to label the individual as "materialistic". The need for a specific object or item is rarely about the object. It is usually about *what the object represents*. It is unlikely that Bennett's (1980) survey respondents were all hoarding and selfish materialists. In describing their needs for their personal possessions, they were revealing their needs to have symbols around them to proclaim (and remind them) that they are: loved, valued, competent, accomplished.... [These terms sound like descriptors from Maslow's (1970) hierarchy, don't they?] In pointing out the importance of personal possessions,

Bennett's survey participants were describing their need for signs that their lives had been fulfilled. Maslow might describe the possessions as reminders that one's needs have been satisfied in life. In a previous paragraph, I described a customized activity for an elderly lady who restored a family heirloom (Seifert, 2000). It was a reminder of her married life and of the happy years with her (late) husband during which they had raised their family. In 2004, Mindy Baker and I described the case of a lady with AD who had cherished a specific religious symbol: a cross. It appeared to provide a cue for prayer, and holding it was soothing to her (Seifert & Baker, 2004; see also, Vance, 2004).

Some recent research via the Chicago Health, Aging, and Social Relations Study (CHASRS; see Cacioppo, Hawkley, Rickett, & Masi, 2005) indicates that physical health and self-esteem are both intricately related to people's social "connectedness".[19] A person's feeling of life's meaning, Cacioppo et al. argued, can be linked to three aspects of the social self. They are one's sense of isolation, his/her perception of social connections via relationships, and an impression of connectedness to groups through voluntary participation in them (my paraphrase of their categories; Cacioppo et al., p. 146). According to CHASRS scientists, personal meaning can be predicted from an individual's sense of his/her "intimate, relational, and collective connectedness" (p. 153). Their results are somewhat consistent with data from a longitudinal study conducted in Spain in which one's feelings of usefulness in the lives of family had a protective effect from cognitive declines up to age 95 (SOLIDAGE study; Beland, Zunzunegui, Alvarado, Otero, & del Ser, 2005). Not only does our connectedness help us to make meaning in life, but it appears to have protective effects against cognitive decline in late life! Thus, we return to my beginning point from Chapter 1. *Every person needs to feel that his/her life is valued—that it has meaning. A sense of purpose can improve life in many ways.*

Via Bennett's (1980) report, possessions can serve as reminders of the meaning one has constructed in his/her life, and results from the CHASRS and SOLIDAGE studies of aging indicate that feelings about social connections can influence many dimensions of life, such as, self-esteem, perceptions of purpose, and even one's cognitive skills (Cacioppo et al., 2005; Beland et al, 2005). Loosely construed, both studies' findings are consistent with Van Boven's (2005) conclusion about happiness. He observed that discretionary money spent on life experiences seems to bring higher reported happiness than discretionary money spent on material possessions. I'll suggest, then, that later in adulthood, a memento—while a material possession—might be valuable as a prop to help a person tell a story from his/her life experience. Moreover, "greater 'story value' of experiences will foster social relationships" (Van Boven, p. 139). *My approach to eldercare is informed by these studies; people want to feel valued, and their social connections and possessions can be important aspects of their sense of worth. When I listen to an elder describe his time in Europe during World War II, when I sit down and look at his service photo and medals, and when I take time to cultivate social connectedness with him in a conversation about his WWII experiences, then I am contributing to his sense of personal value.*

3

Individual Differences in Perception

Humans are not rocks. We sense. We take in information through sounds, views, and other modalities. What's more, people display a wide array of interpretations and reactions to the same information. Yes, we do sense. And we also *think*. We interpret what we have sensed.

For fifteen years, I have taught college courses related to human "sensation" and "perception". Those two words are used interchangeably in everyday conversation, but scientists do not treat them as synonyms. "Sensations" involve registration of incoming information at the ears; eyes; taste buds; olfactory (nasal) membranes; and skin or body "sensors" (see Goldstein, 2004; Gregory, 1966). "Perceptions" are *interpretations* of sensory input. Philosopher David Hume (see Hergenhahn & Olsen, 1997, pp. 36-37) contrasted an "impression" with an "idea", respectively. The former involves physical registration of incoming information, and the latter represents an individual's mind acting on information in order to understand it and build associations to it. Hume argued (reminiscent of Plato's writing) that a person cannot know anything with absolute sureness, because all ideas are based on [subjective] interpretations of reality.

Have you ever looked at the dashboard of your car on a very sunny day? The polymer coating on most dashboards causes incredible glare on a bright day—so much so that, despite its color, the dash appears almost white. But when you look at it, you probably don't gasp with astonishment and shriek, "Oh, it's an incredible miracle! My dashboard has turned white. Call the newspaper!!!!!" No. In fact, you probably still think of the dash in terms of its "actual" hue. In that scenario, your sensation changes due to fluctuating lighting, but your perception remains stable. Your mental interpretation of the dashboard's color stays the same, regardless of whether it is a bright day or an overcast day—presumably because your experience tells you a lot about how lighting conditions can change the appearance of things. Thus, the color's appearance remains stable in different lighting situations.

When you are at the mall with a friend, you might plan to separate for a few minutes, because she wants to go to a store in the next corridor. You say, "OK. I'm going into this store. Let's meet back here in about 15 minutes." And off she goes—walking away from you. As she heads down the mall-way, you are unlikely to panic and scream, "Oh, no! My friend is shrinking! Get help!!!!" Of course you don't. Even though the visual sensation (via the image that is projected onto the retina of your eye) of your shopping buddy is shrinking as she walks away, your perception is that she is walking away and NOT getting smaller. Your perception can be stable, even though your sensations change.

Several years ago, my husband and I were on vacation. We had been driving for hours and were both bleary-eyed. We were in a very flat geographic area with which we were unfamiliar. Judging distances across the plain was difficult for us, because we both grew up in the hilly, glaciated Great Lakes region of the USA. Here we were: exhausted and approaching an exit ramp which extended for at least .5 mile. As we continued traveling on the main highway, another car headed down the ramp, so that it was situated to the right of our car, but quite far away. My husband, fatigued and unfamiliar with the landscape, was startled by the sudden appearance of this car in his right peripheral (side) view. To his tired brain, it seemed as if there was a tiny matchbox car floating in space within inches of his right eye—rather than the actual-sized car that was almost .25 mile away from us on the ramp. He looked quickly to his right. Startled—he said, "Was something floating or flying around by my right eye? ...Oh, I see. There's a car over on that exit ramp."

Obviously, we decided to stop at the next exit and rest for a while before continuing on our trip! But the incident provides an excellent example of how much humans depend on interpretations of everyday sensory experiences. When our "powers of interpretation" break down due to fatigue, degraded lighting, illness, or unfamiliarity with a stimulus event, then we can be left puzzled and bewildered. Visual illusions and magic take advantage of those types of circumstances. Magicians know that it is possible to cause a "disconnect" between what is sensed and how it is interpreted, and they take full advantage of it.

You might wonder why I decided to discuss perceptual illusions in a book about caring for senior citizens. It's simple. All humans are susceptible to varied perceptual experiences and illusions—elders, too. When an aging sensory system or a disease interferes with perceptual interpretations, one can be left stunned, confused, or afraid of the perceived stimulus.

Consider facial expressions. Paul Ekman (2003) has spent his career studying human facial expressions. He reported convincing evidence that several facial expressions (corresponding to emotions like happiness and sadness) are inborn in humans. His studies of the

Fore people of New Guinea were an incredible beginning to a distinguished research career on emotion-linked facial gestures, and his book *Emotions Revealed* is a very readable review of his work and conclusions. Ekman has described and illustrated (with photographs of his "physiognomically-gifted" daughter, Eve) some basic human emotions through facial gestures for happiness, sadness, anger, disgust, fear, and surprise (with the last two sometimes proving difficult to discriminate from each other).

A reader might also wonder why I've chosen to initiate a conversation about emotion in the current chapter—when I have already indicated that a later chapter of this volume will cover issues about eldercare and emotions. The answer is simple: perception of others is one of the most critical parts of human life. Yet, there are amazing differences between individuals with respect to *how* we perceive events, things, ourselves and each other (again, reflecting on Hume's assertion that human ideas are *necessarily* biased interpretations of sensory experiences).

Facial expressions seem to be a key part of perception and action. We watch others; we react. They watch us; they, in turn, react, and so on. Even scientists who disagree with Ekman (2003)—about the link between internal experiences of emotion and expressions on the human face—do concede that facial expressions can help us predict another person's upcoming behavior (e.g., an opinion attributed to Campos by Azar, 2000; for original work see Campos, Frankel, & Camras, 2004). Facial expressions serve as cues to what someone might do or say next.

Even if they disagree about *why* it is true, scientists agree that facial expressions are critical in human life (Ekman, 2003; Campos et al., 2004).[1] It follows, logically, that they are critical in the lives of elders, too. However, facial expressions can be misperceived (see Ekman's work for information about micro-expressions, mixed expressions, and deceptive expressions). Humans use tacit, innate knowledge about expressions of emotion, and individuals also use their own experiences to judge expressions as honest or as disingenuous (fake or deceitful). In the language of psychology: An actor's expression (with "actor" being just another term for the person engaging in a specific behavior) can be misunderstood by an observer (i.e., the person who sees the expression). Here is my story about face perception...

I have a BIG smile. What can I say? I love life. As my Grammy used to say about me, "She knows who she is. She was *born* knowing it!" The story of my thoughts is written on my face. I have a sallow, Sicilian-

American complexion with lots of yellow undertones and very dark features (dark brown eyes, dark hair, and very pronounced eyebrows). When I smile, lots of teeth show and my arched, black eyebrows are a HUGE feature of my smiling face. Here's the glitch: that arched, raised eyebrows are not a typical feature of a genuine smile—even though they are *always* a part of my face (happy, sad, or otherwise!).

When I am providing eldercare, I smile a lot. But to some observers—especially individuals with AD, who sometimes experience paranoia and diminished cognitive skills in managing their emotional reactions—my smile can seem like an "over-smile" (or an attempt to make a smile when I'm not really feeling happy). The big arched eyebrows may seem more like a sinister attempt at a disingenuous smile to someone who doesn't know me. On more than one occasion, I've observed an individual with Alzheimer-type dementia to raise his/her eyebrows in surprise as s/he fixates on my eyebrows. [You can often notice *where* someone is fixating on your face, if you are close enough to follow his/her gaze.] Here I confront the very issue of individual differences in perception, because I must sometimes "tone down" my real smile, so that I don't scare or alarm the people for whom I help provide care. To one person, my smile might seem like a gleeful expression, but for another, it might seem menacing or ominous.

Living around other people, we confront an important principle: that there's no disputing taste ("de gustibus non est disputandum" an ancient Roman aphorism). Antecedent to that: when two people *sense* the same thing, they might experience different *perceptual interpretations* (and a different affinity or disdain for the object that is perceived). [Indeed, it's those different interpretations of an event that so often lead to the 'taste disputes'.] While it is the case that one person's perception might be closer to objective reality than someone else's, it can be extremely difficult to prove it! The philosopher Nietzsche wrote, "...you tell me...that there is no disputing taste and tasting? But all life is a dispute over taste...." (Nietzsche, 1883/1967). Presumably, if human perceptions were uniform, then there would be no arguments about them.

People disagree about what they have perceived, and they haggle about what *really* happened. It is very difficult to debate someone's perception, but people do it anyway! In the USA, court cases are built on these very types of controversies: that one witness reported X and another witness observed Y. Disputing someone else's perception is often fruitless, and in eldercare this is doubly true (probably because we are much less experienced at the debate than many of our elders!). I once saw a T-shirt with the words, "Age and treachery will triumph over youth and vitality." [2] One way to *reframe* the quote *in favor of elders* is that: "Age and wisdom will triumph over youth's indiscretions." To argue with another person about differing perceptions can be futile. A sample case is the caregiver who tries to "correct" the misperceptions of a person with AD—with the result being an argument or a catastrophic reaction (e.g., physical violence by the person with AD) *without* bringing him/her around to the caregiver's viewpoint.

About my BIG smile, I could go around all day saying, "Now, I'm really happy. This is my *real* smile!" But how far would that get me? What about the individual who has moderate-to-severe dementia? How can I convince him or her that my "over-smile" is genuine? The answer is, "Not likely!!!!" And what is my motivation? It would seem that I want people to accept me as I am and to take my smile as genuine. I want people to *accept me as I am, so that I know I have value. If this is true, then I can begin by accepting them and valuing them. I should value their perceptions and opinions. If I disagree with them, perhaps I might at least consider a little tolerance?* If an individual with right hemisphere stroke or Alzheimer-type dementia has difficulty interpreting my big smile, then I can show that

I care for him/her by toning down my toothy grin and saying words that convey my sentiments. I might smile softly and say, "Hi, [resident's name]. How are you today? Your dress is very pretty. The blue flowers bring out the blue in your eyes!" My words convey a tone of caring that reinforces the genuineness of my smile. My words are selected on the basis of my knowledge about the specific person whom I address. If I know a gentleman likes to follow a specific sports team, I might smile and ask, "[His name], how are you? Your [name of team] really walloped the other team last night! Did you give them some coaching advice?" When we consider perception, we recognize the importance of impression management in our interpersonal interactions.

Impression management is very much about how we wish to be perceived by other people. It also includes the ways that people's reactions to us shape our self-perceptions. Charles Horton Cooley (see Szacki, 1976) used 'looking-glass self' to label this *molding of self-perception through interpersonal interactions*. The principle is simple. When we behave in particular ways, we are given feedback from other people about whether our actions "fit in". We use that information to adjust our future behaviors: either away from, or toward the expected outcomes. If the behaviors expected of us by the group do not fit our goals or expectations, then we might: 1) try to change the group expectations and rules, or 2) leave the group to find one that better fits our goals and perceptions (see Sternberg, 1997; Goleman, 2002; Bolt, 2004). Over time, we strive to behave in ways that reflect *the person we want to be.* Part of this process involves impression management—whereby we try to *appear* in a particular way in our social life. We act on the world, and then we process feedback from the people around us. Did they like what I did? Do they approve of me? The feedback can reward or punish; it tells us whether our intended messages have been received.

When I work with elders, I observe that there are some individuals who love the role of "grandparent". In fact, these are folks who are called "Grandma" or "Grandpa" by many (regardless of family relationship). They *want* to be perceived in such a role, and they look for opportunities to appear "grand-parental". Over the years, I have met many residents in long-term care who would be willing to comply with any wish I might express (e.g., to prepare for a meal, to groom, to prepare for bed)—as long as I acknowledged one of their ideal roles (like "grandparent"). When I call someone by the label "Grandma", I reinforce her looking-glass concept of self-as-grandparent. If she enjoys that role, then my label might serve as a reward that reinforces her positive self-concept (Szacki, 1976). You might ask: 1) "Is that ethical?" Or, 2) "Is such a person cognitively intact? Doesn't she know that she isn't your grandmother?" For many senior citizens, the answers are "yes". They know everyone around them isn't necessarily a "grandchild". However, they love the role of grandparent and prefer to be perceived in that role. Still other elders prefer the parent role, and some like the spousal role or a certain professional role.[3] *When we relate to people in ways that indicate respect for their preferred roles, then we honor their sense of self and contribute to their sense of their own value.*

You marvel, "How can I relate to someone who prefers his or her role as spouse? I can't very well pretend to be married to him/her!" No, and in the case of the grandparent role, too, you might not feel comfortable calling people your grandparents when they are not. However, you can honor someone's desired role. You can honor him or her as *someone's* spouse or as *someone's* grandparent. For many elderly women, dozens of years might be spent in widowhood, and reminiscing about those years as someone's spouse can bring great joy. I have spent time in conversation with many widows and widowers who enjoy telling me about their years of "wedded adventure". They might share stories about their life as a couple, their trials during war years, their hardships as they raised a family, and their great happiness about the harvest of many years' hard work together. As they reminisce, they can slip back into that treasured role of spouse (or parent), and their stories can help them to demonstrate how they have been valued and how they have created meaning in their lives. Similarly, someone who valued his/her role in the work force can be prompted to reminisce about it, or s/he can be asked to use skills in volunteer activities that derive specifically from work-related expertise.

I was once acquainted with a very special woman who had been a nurse for fifty years. She provided us with a wealth of knowledge about health and pediatric care, and many of us would consult with her for advice about our children's nutrition, vaccinations, "ouchies", and developmental milestones. We benefited from her wisdom, and the "consultations" helped her to maintain an identity in one of her most valued roles in life. *When you identify and acknowledge the most valued roles of people for whom you provide care, then you can honor them in those roles.*

When I engage in conversation with an elder who has Alzheimer's disease (or an associated condition), I promote orientation by cueing memories and thoughts about his/her valued roles. However, I try to do so in careful ways that encourage a person, without prompting sorrow or anger. For example, I follow the individual's lead in a conversation, rather than forging ahead on my own. This prevents me from startling someone with an undesirable topic. I would be unlikely to start talking about someone's deceased spouse without a verbal or behavioral prompt. If a spouse is mentioned, I might say, "[Listener's name], remind me. In what year were the two of you married?" Notice that the question asks about an established fact, and it can orient the person in time (because I've used a past tense verb). For an individual with cognitive decline or dementia, the mere use of the past tense verb can gently remind him or her that the wedding is a *past* event. My further interest is expressed and orientation to time is cued with another question like, "And for how many years were the two of you married?" Again, I allow the elder to lead conversation topics, because grieving and reminiscing can be flip-sides of the same coin (see Manning, 1991). I want to encourage the latter, without prompting painful grief to resurface on every occurrence of reminiscing.[4]

Facial expressions, emotions, and social cues are important parts of adult life. However, perception and aging are about more than facial expressions and person perceptions. [In Chapter 5, on emotion, I'll have more to say about Ekman's (2003) research and person perception.] For many aging adults, the senses give "wrong" information. As I mentioned earlier, aging can change the senses. In turn, perceptions of people, places, and events might be altered. In the foregoing section, I described some issues related to perception of people. In the upcoming application section, I will address some aspects of aging that relate to one's perception of environment and to the design of living spaces for eldercare.

Application: Environment and Design in Eldercare

There are lots of books and articles about eldercare improvement through architectural and environmental design (e.g., Bennett, 1980; Regnier, 1997; Percival, 2002; Barnes et al., 2002; Morgan & Stewart, 2000). I don't plan to describe all the elements of environmental design for eldercare in this brief section. However, I will point to some of the critical aspects of design that might interact with elders' sensations, perceptions, and actions. Many of these points include considerations of the changes in aging sensory systems. Some of them derive from my specific experiences in eldercare research. For still others, I refer you to your own state and local guidelines for day-, group-, and long-term care, because many states and municipalities have considered the safety of special-needs and eldercare environments in determining licensure for those types of facilities (e.g., widths of corridors and doorways; wheelchair accessibility; and natural lighting to improve affect/mood, sleep-wake cycles, and glare problems).

Overall, there are many different techniques to improve the quality of life and comfort in eldercare settings. Bennett (1980) and others (e.g., Willcocks, Peace, & Kellaher, 1987) have described some important aspects of elder life, which include having one's own possessions, having privacy, and having an environment that promotes safety (with excellent lighting, reduced glare, diminished foul odors, and "landmarks" that promote "wayfinding"; Barnes et al., 2002; Passini, Pigot, Rainville, & Tetreault, 2000). Regnier (1997) stressed the importance of soliciting residents' opinions about design elements in long-term care (although I dispute his tendency to discount staff opinions). Barnes et al. (2002) emphasized the study of building *uses* in concert with facility design, and Zeisel et al. (2003) devised an "E-B" (environment-behavior) factor model for predicting desirable design features of residential units for dementia care. Aesthetics and function must be taken together, because they both affect quality of life in eldercare. Overall, we must consider the needs of elders (i.e., for physical care, for safety, to feel loved/accepted, to feel worthwhile, and to feel that they have the potential for success in their endeavors; Maslow, 1970; see also, Greenspan & Wieder, 1998; Percival, 2002; Bennett). When we consider the elements of design as critical to life's meaning and quality, then we begin to understand the importance of elders' perceptions of their environment.

As I described earlier, the senses change with aging. For individuals with aging vision, glare is increased and vision is yellowed. This can diminish a person's ability to judge a surface as wet or dry. An elder might be capable of reasoning to solve the glare illusion, but might not possess the agility or mobility required to test the assumption. As one gentleman put it, "I think that shiny tile floor is probably dry, but I'm not willing to risk a broken hip to prove it!" His physical body might be aging, but he can reason his way out of many potentially dangerous predicaments.

Another individual might have Alzheimer-type dementia, and the glare illusion might be compounded by an inability to use logic to over-ride the perception of a wet floor. A nurse's aid might say, "Don't worry. The floor is dry. It's just shiny." However, a person with cognitive decline might still refuse to walk on, or to be wheeled onto, such a floor, because the glossy surface *looks* wet and slippery. The words of reassurance about its safety are soon forgotten, but the actual semblance of the floor as wet persists! It's also a common occurrence for a caregiver to encounter resistance from a person with dementia when moving along any transition in flooring in *either* direction (that is, either onto it or off of it). Someone might refuse to walk from carpet to tile floor *or vice versa*, because s/he perceives any flooring transition as a visual cliff (a drop-off). Interpreting changes in the surface of a floor or an object is a learned talent [see E. Gibson's (1969) work on perceptual development].[5] With aging senses *and* dementia, a person might be unable to discern that the apparent visual cliff and the glare illusion are not veridical perceptions (i.e., not reality). With diminished capacity to assess the floor's risk, the individual with dementia might routinely refuse to venture out onto it. If the tile floor is en route to the dining hall or bath house, then the appearance of the flooring can produce an undesirable effect: with the individual who has dementia rejecting invitations to go to dinner or to have a shower.

For situations that involve glare or visual cliff illusions there are some simple solutions. First, *know your needs*. Establish a goal that is related to them. Do you need to improve traffic? Or is the goal to stop traffic (like halting exits from a dementia care unit)? If the current type of flooring impedes traffic by causing falls or by making able elders wary of locations where they *should* walk, then diminish the appearance of glare by reducing the shine on a floor. Be careful not to merely cut floor shine by letting wax build up. Old wax on a floor can become dull and tacky, and a sticky floor boosts foot-to-floor friction. It can catch rubber shoe soles and increase the likelihood of tripping. Instead of floors that need high shine and that let wax build up, consider flooring options that have little shine, are not slippery, and that are also not likely to become sticky or tacky when left without wax. There are experts in engineering who can provide more advice about slip resistance and flooring (see Burnfield & Powers, 2006). I did see a beautiful floor recently that was tile, with the appearance of wood. It was washable, but the resultant look was not glossy or slick to foot traffic (Burnfield, Tsai, & Powers, 2005; Cham & Redfern, 2002).

To Increase Desirable Traffic

Visual cliffs appear when there are transitions in floor texture, depth, or color. If *desirable* traffic is being stopped by flooring transitions, then reduce the number of areas where flooring changes occur (e.g., from carpet to tile) and eliminate transitions which involve changes in texture or depth. Because of the increased risk of falling down or tripping among elderly people

(Whitbourne, 2001, p. 105; see DiGiovanna, 1994, Ch. 8 & Ch. 9), it is important to decrease the number of transitions from one type of flooring to another. If transitions must occur, then the border (e.g., from pile carpet to a lower tile floor) should be well lighted and marked with a large, printed sign (like "STEP DOWN"; with black print on a bright yellow background being one of the most noticeable contrast combinations). If you're using visual patterns to show contrast (e.g., wallpaper patterns or tile patterns with hue-on-hue contrasts), then green shades tend to reveal the most overall pattern contrast and yellow hues seem to reveal the least (with blues and reds showing intermediate pattern contrast; Hegde & Woodson, 1999). Each environment is different, and individuals who reside there have specific needs. Thus, it is impossible for me to give advice to fit every situation. Generally, though, it is better to reduce transitions of depth, texture, or color of flooring when a surface is continuous (i.e., having no steps up or down)—especially in areas that must be traveled frequently by elders.

The converse case occurs when there must be flooring transitions (like steps, bumps, or unevenness).

Then it is advisable to create a very noticeable visual cliff via a color transition, because this will increase the probability that travelers will notice the flooring transition and will not trip at one that is unmarked (or unnoticeable). I have noticed many cases in which padded carpet makes a transition down to thin tile. Decorators can *accentuate the visual cliff* by using a very different color and shade of tile than carpet. One example I particularly prefer is light grayish-blue carpet with a transition to deep burgundy-red tile. This makes the visual cliff more visible for well elders who must traverse the area. Paired with a sign (e.g., "STEP DOWN"; "STEP UP"), the transition is more likely to be noticed and less likely to precipitate tripping. Realize, though, that elders may become shy of these "cliffs" and avoid them (for fear of falling). Overall, for physically fit, cognitively intact elders, it is better to minimize unevenness in flooring.[6] This makes "trip-free travel" more likely for them. When steps impede handicapped-accessibility, consider the use of a gently sloping ramp (and not a steeply inclined one), and work with a licensed architect who has experience designing gerontological environments. Finally, *do* place grip bars or hand rails at appropriate heights so that elders can steady themselves by holding on as they walk (Zukerman, 2003).

To Decrease Undesirable Traffic

For senior citizens with dementia, glare and flooring transitions can be utilized to *discourage* traffic out of exits, into other residents' rooms, or into dangerous areas. A dramatic transition [for example, from lighter blue-gray carpet to a darker, glossy (shiny, yet not slippery) black tile floor] can greatly decrease traffic, because an individual with dementia might perceive the transition as a very deep step (via the illusion of the drop-off from the carpet to the tile) or as wet tile (as in the transition from carpet to a high gloss tile floor that is not wet). Many eldercare facilities use glare and visual illusions effectively to discourage wandering into unsafe areas (see Zukerman, 2003, p. 261). Warner (2000) provided some useful advice for caregivers at home. In particular, he made the point that a visual cliff should cover a wide enough section of floor to deter any urge to "jump over it" (see Warner, p. 105; p. 276). Otherwise, its purpose (i.e., as a passive barrier) is defeated, and the individual with dementia might simply hop across it to the other side!

In some cases, wall coverings can be used to camouflage exits, and I saw an especially successful design in a group home for individuals with mild-to-moderate dementia. It was a wall of tasteful wooden panels that appeared to be solid (like wainscoting). However, the middle panel was a push-able door that opened into a small anteroom near one of the building's exits. The "trompe l'oile" design (pronounced "trump loy": an art term meaning "tricks the eye") was effective as camouflage, and residents rarely approached the area to attempt an exit.[7] Flooring and wall coverings can be used to create a home-like, non-institutional atmosphere (Regnier, 1997). Moreover, they can be used to improve or discourage traffic by considering the influences of aging vision, mobility, and special conditions (such as AD or other dementia) on perceptions of design (Mayer & Darby, 1991; Kincaid & Peacock, 2003; Zeisel et al., 2003).

No matter how we assess environment, the reality of elder life is that context design can greatly impact its functionality. Overall, it is important to evaluate a person's needs and construct (or renovate) the environment to foster better quality of life and optimal functioning. Bennett's (1980) conclusion is long-standing: that *context is critical for the quality of elder life.*

4

Thinking and Memory in Older Adulthood

"Cognitive aging" is a specialty area in gerontology. In it, we study age-related differences and changes in learning, remembering, solving problems, and one's intelligence. The scientific literature is immense and covers questions such as whether comparisons of younger and older adults are affected by age, cohort (an approximately six-year interval around one's birth year during which peers are born), generation (an interval larger than a cohort in which individuals experience "history" together), physiology, and personal experience. Another issue is whether comparisons of younger and older adults are even relevant (i.e., perhaps being comparisons of human conditions that are so different as to be like contrasting apples with oranges).

Although some research indicated declines in several key cognitive skills as people age (see Schaie, 1996), there is evidence that part of the documented effect is due to "cross-sectional" comparison (i.e., testing people who are different ages at just one point in time, like 20- and 60-year-olds in 2008). A single comparison of intelligence, thinking, or memory across several age groups who are tested just once can suffer from several problems. In such a study, age can be confounded with (an expression that means "mixed up with" or "entangled with") one's cohort and generation. If we conducted a study of memory and tested 20-year-olds, 40-year-olds, and 60-year-olds, we would be studying three different generations of people. Thus, any memory differences we observed might be related to participants' ages (suggesting an effect of aging on memory), or they might be due to the different histories of the groups (possibly indicating that one's birth during or just after World War II had a different effect than birth during the Vietnam War or birth just before the Cold War ended). There are so many *different* events that happen in history, it would be difficult to determine how historical events had affected the groups differently and whether those effects might have interacted with aging.

Because of problematic age-by-age comparisons in cross-sectional research designs, many researchers have adopted different strategies for investigating age differences. An alternative method is "longitudinal research" which follows one set of individuals over time. Because the same participants are tested and later re-tested, the influences of history on research participants are more likely to be uniform (or at least similar). If a researcher tested and later re-tested people born in the

U.S. during the Korean War, it would be reasonable to assume that many of the influences of that war era on those persons would be similar. Effects of public policies, educational techniques, and the "Zeitgeist" (the "spirit" or "mood" of an era in history) on all those participants would be presumably comparable. Unfortunately, a drawback of the simple, longitudinal approach is that some effects can vary systematically with history. For example, individuals who are all born around the same time might experience history similarly. They might also be taught similarly (e.g., with emphasis on one set of skills rather than another). As a result, observed changes among the set of persons in a longitudinal study might be due as much to the specific ways those persons have been taught, trained, occupied, or employed, as they are to real aging-related changes (Bee & Boyd, 2002). Researchers talk about these "history effects" as serious concerns in longitudinal research. This type of effect has been observed by Schaie (1996) in relation to number skills—for which older cohorts performed better (those born in 1910, 1917, and 1924) when the effects of practice and response rate were removed statistically (see Figure 12-7, p. 368, Schaie & Willis, 2002).

A partial solution to problems inherent in cross-sectional and longitudinal research is to adopt a sequential approach (see Schaie's "Most Efficient Design", Schaie & Willis, 2002, pp. 116-120). The optimal form of sequential design combines the former two methods by following at least two different age groups over time. Thus, it yields two or more comparisons of the groups *over time.* It also adds younger cohorts as time passes. In this way, the effects of cohort or generation can be separated from mere effects of time passing (related to aging; Schaie & Willis, p. 117). If similar trends are observed over time and across groups, it indicates that age-related changes—rather than cohort differences—are critical to those trends (see Bee & Boyd, 2002; Schaie & Willis, 2002). One of the most well-known studies of this type is the Seattle Longitudinal Study (which has included aspects of both longitudinal and cross-sectional techniques; Schaie, 1996).

A key result of the Seattle Longitudinal Study has been to eschew the myth that mental abilities generally decline with age. That myth seems to have been largely an artifact of cohort and generation differences in earlier cross-sectional studies (Schaie & Willis, 2002; Schaie, 1996). Indeed, much of what was observed in earlier cross-sectional studies most likely stemmed from cohort differences in particular skills (like spatial skills and inductive reasoning; see Schaie).

Cohort differences might have been misinterpreted by some researchers as actual cognitive declines associated with aging. As I mentioned in the previous paragraph, many apparent differences in cognitive abilities might be due to differences in education, training, employment and other factors across cohorts and generations. For instance, opportunities for high-school education (and beyond) have greatly improved in the USA over the past century (see Ronnlund, Nyberg, Backman, & Nilsson, 2005).

The effects of aging on reasoning and memory have been studied in various ways. The reader might recall an aphorism, "You can't teach an old dog new tricks" (as referenced by Brewer, 1898). Besides being a pejorative (insulting) expression, overall, it is untrue. Many older adults learn new sports, activities, jobs, and games successfully (Whitbourne, 2001; Rowe & Kahn, 1998). Rabbitt, Diggle, Smith, Holland, and McInnes (2001) reported that older adults performed less well than younger adults on a test of fluid abilities (which are generally associated with episodic memory; see Ronnlund, Nyberg, Backman, & Nilsson, 2005), but they also reported that elders benefited more than younger adults from practice due to repeated administration of the test [i.e., AH4 (1) given at intervals of 24 or 36 months; Rabbitt et al.].

Ronnlund et al. (2005; see their Figures 5 and 6) analyzed a cohort-matched sample in order to help them rule out practice effects and education effects. In addition, they used both cross-sectional and longitudinal approaches to reveal no diminishment of episodic memory before 60 years-of-age, with some deterioration thereafter. With respect to semantic memory, they observed slight improvement with age (i.e., up to about 55 years), with a slight decrease after age 55. It appears that a person's highest level of education is an important predictor of cognitive function in older adulthood, with individuals maintaining higher cognitive function longer if they have achieved a higher level of education, overall (Schaie & Willis, 2002; see Rabbitt et al., 2001, Table 1; Ronnlund et al.). There are many reasons this might be true, including the high cognitive demands of professions that require more education. If an individual works, for example, as an attorney, there are high demands to recall facts about cases on a regular basis. The individual is, in essence, "exercising" memory as s/he remembers cases, rulings, and precedents. If such a person were to participate in a research study about age differences in fact based memory, s/he could have an advantage over someone who works in a job that emphasizes different skills (like sensorimotor coordination—which probably would not have the same beneficial transfer of practice into a study of fact based memory skills). Alternatively, in a study of spatial skills, someone who has spent his/her time rebuilding carburetors might out-perform someone who has devoted his/her career to bookkeeping. Much of the issue is what you practice and whether you're tested on it!

Given the added benefit of practice for elders, it might not be surprising to learn that older participants can benefit from training to enhance memory strategies (Camp, 1999; Camp, Foss, O'Hanlon, & Stevens, 1996). Camp and his colleagues have reported several results over the years to indicate that practice can benefit older adults—even individuals with Alzheimer-type dementia. In a training paradigm that used spaced practice (see Landauer & Bjork, 1978, for more about the scientific basis of spaced-retrieval) and a daily calendar, individuals with dementia and their caregivers were trained to use the calendar to cue functional behaviors (e.g., bathing, grooming, eating, taking medications). Training consisted of once-a-week sessions in which the participant was asked, "How are you going to remember what to do each day?" (Camp et al., 1996, p. 203). For individuals with dementia, training begins at a retrieval interval of 0 seconds. That is, the question is asked and answered by the trainer until the participant can successfully answer the query with, "Look at my calendar" (also p. 203). Then, the question is asked after 20 seconds. If the participant successfully responds, then the retrieval interval is extended to 40 seconds—after which the question is asked again, and so on (with intervals increasing from 40 to 60, from 60 to 90, from 90 to 120, and from 120 to 150 seconds, after successive correct responses). If a failure occurs, then the retrieval interval reverts to the most recent successful interval (a success at 60 seconds with a failure at 90 would lead the trainer to revert to the 60-second question-response interval until the participant had successfully responded; Camp et al.).

The technique of spaced-retrieval described above can be conceptualized as the minimalist's distributed practice paradigm (after 0, 20, 40, 60 seconds, etc.), and it can be utilized to train adults who have short-term memory problems. A similar technique can help children—who, generally, have short-term memory inferior to that of normal adults—to remember tasks (about repetition priming and infants, see Bearce & Rovee-Collier, 2006; for memory training and elementary school-aged children, see Still, 2005). The casual reader, however, should not dismiss spaced-retrieval as fit only for young children and individuals with dementia. The basic technique is one that typical adults naturally use (such as repeating a phone number to oneself while putting down the phone book and reaching for the phone, or rehearsing directions from a cookbook while walking across the kitchen to pull the needed ingredients from a cupboard). It's a usual activity of normal adult memory to engage in techniques for remembering: like simple rehearsal through repetition and like more elaborate rehearsal (e.g., making an acronym out of a shopping list, so that one can more easily remember the items to be purchased). Camp et al. (1996) adapted this naturally occurring rehearsal effect to aid remembering by persons who experience memory difficulties. The general method of spaced rehearsal is appropriate for just about anyone, and for many of us, the intervals can be spaced farther apart for even better results (see Bahrick & Hall, 2005, who cited 14- and 30-day rehearsal intervals as superior to single-day spaced practice for normal functioning young adults).

Bahrick and Hall (2005) pointed out that for normal memory, spacing rehearsal far enough apart to identify those items that are worst-remembered in a list can actually lead to better overall memory for material, because an individual can identify and pay closer attention to rehearsal of the most troublesome items. I saw this effect in real life one semester when I was trying to memorize the names of about forty students in my introductory psychology class. I hadn't realized that I wasn't correctly remembering the names and faces of two students who were best friends and who always sat together in class. After we had a long weekend, I called on one of them with the other's name. After that, I paid deliberate attention to rehearsing their correct names while looking at their photos in the college student directory. Had the long weekend not occurred, and had I not had the break from tri-weekly rehearsal of student names via role call, I probably wouldn't have realized that I *didn't know* which best friend possessed each of the two first names.

In a traditional spaced-retrieval memory task, it's all about successively increasing the time between sessions of rehearsal. Overall, this can lead to more robust memory for practiced information (Landauer & Bjork, 1978)! For one person, successively increasing intervals from 0 seconds (with increasing intervals to 20, 40, 60 seconds and beyond; as in the study by Camp et al., 1996) might be appropriate. For another individual an initial interval of 2 minutes might work. And a third learner might need only two "rehearsals", spaced 30 minutes apart, in order to remember that s/he must go to a doctor's appointment the next morning at 10:00 AM. There are individual differences in the spacing of and number of retrievals required to successfully rehearse and remember a piece of information. In a spaced remembering activity, it's key to know: 1) how long to wait before asking, and 2) how often to ask about a critical piece of to-be-remembered information.

Application: Memory Lags
and Prompts

For someone who has a normal memory, learning a list of new people (e.g., faces and names of people at your new workplace) might be as simple as repeating a person's name after being introduced to him or her. Then, after a minute or so, you might rehearse it by thinking, "His name is Jack." After having a brief conversation with the person, you might rehearse again by saying, "Well, it has been very nice to meet you, Jack." The next day, when you see the person, rehearse again by greeting him, "Hi, Jack. How are you today?" If Jack is a person you don't work with directly, you might only see him once per day (e.g., in the lunch room). If you deliberately rehearse people's names (like Jack's) by greeting people each day as you see them, then this should lead to better long-term memories for their names. After a time, you should be able to defer retrieval of names to more distant intervals (e.g., greeting Jack every 14th day). At the longer delay, you should be able to better pinpoint those names and faces that are giving you trouble, and then you can put extra effort into memorizing them. Notice, that my example is tailored to fit the research on practice that we see in the scientific literature (e.g., Bahrick & Hall, 2005). However, in everyday life you might encounter social demands to greet people (and therefore rehearse their names) more often. After all, it might seem odd to say to someone, "I'm sorry, but I can't greet you with your name today, because I'm trying to wait 14 days to discover whether your name is one of the better-remembered or worst-remembered ones in my memory!" [Then, again, some folks won't necessarily notice whether you've greeted them by name or not. Conversely, while this is a great exercise for people with normal memories, it's really not a way to treat those for whom you provide eldercare: who should be addressed by name in order to honor their person-hood and to bring their attention to you.]

For people who have memory difficulties (e.g., because of AD or a related type of dementia), it might be useful to start with very brief rehearsal intervals (as suggested by Camp and his colleagues; Camp et al., 1996; Bourgeois et al., 2003). As I mentioned in a previous paragraph, starting with rehearsal after 20 seconds and increasing intervals by 20 or by 30 seconds after each successful prompt with correct recall can help the individual with dementia to remember specific pieces of information better!

A *cue hierarchy* can be another useful component of retrieve-to-remember tasks (Camp et al., 1996). On a given trial (i.e., an attempt to remember), a learner purposefully retrieves information with the help of a designated probe. If retrieval fails, then another probe (from a set of progressively more specific ones) can be given. Cued recall provides support for memory rehearsal (Camp et al.; Bourgeois et al., 2003). By creating a cue hierarchy, the "teacher" can be ready with a set of memory cues (ranging from a basic "remember" probe to some very specific cues).

To demonstrate a cue hierarchy, let's take the example of remembering an appointment for a haircut at 9:00 AM. One's alarm clock rings at 7:00 AM, and s/he awakens. For many people, the clock sound cues him/her to think, "Now, what must I accomplish today?" That thought, alone, can cue remembering in a very basic way, "Right. I must go to get my haircut at 9:00 AM!" And with that, retrieval has been successful. This success in recall might not always occur, though. Knowing that we might not recall all the appointments of every day, we make date-books and calendars for ourselves. If I haven't recalled the appointments for today upon asking myself what I have to do, then I can cue remembering by looking at my date-book. For individuals who have normal memory, this might be the general way in which they use cues in order to remember daily appointments.

In some research on the use of cue hierarchies in eldercare, the general format of the cue list is specified by the abbreviation "SPVTI": Semantic, Phonemic, Visual, Tactile, Imitation (Bourgeois et al., 2003, p. 369). The following list provides an example of cueing that is structured with SPVTI:

1) If I want to cue a forgetful elder to look at his or her daily calendar (in order to discover today's appointment at the barbershop), then I begin by probing the meaning of the act: to look at the calendar. I ask, "There is something we need to look at. It lists our appointments."

2) If the individual does not recall that s/he needs to "look at the daily calendar," then we proceed to give a sound cue for the goal, "k" (for "calendar").

3) Further failure to remember calendar checking can be met with a visual cue, as the caregiver points toward the daily calendar.

4) Additional cueing can be provided tactually by handing the daily calendar to the forgetful person. Sometimes, this type of touch-interaction with the to-be-

remembered item can prompt remembering. The elder might say, "Oh, yes. I need to look at the calendar."

5) A final step toward successful remembering—if the tactile cue isn't effective—is imitation: in which the caregiver says, "I look at the daily calendar," while looking at it. The individual who is being cued can then imitate calendar looking (see Bourgeois et al., Section 2.4, after which this example is fashioned).

For persons with dementia (PwD: a general term for individuals who have cognitive impairment), the mental leap from remembering without specific cues to remembering to keep and look at a date-book can be huge. Thus, we might develop a hierarchy of cues for him/her that would bring about remembering. While SPVTI can be useful (Bourgeois et al., 2003), there are some other ways to develop a cue hierarchy. For such a person, we might set the alarm clock for 7:00 AM and ask, "What do you have to do today?" whenever s/he awakens. If the question doesn't prompt remembering, then we might ask, "Do you have any appointments today?" (and thus cue memory by making a specific reference to the fact that s/he might have an outside engagement). If that is an unsuccessful probe, then we might ask him or her to, "Please, look at the calendar (date-book) in order to check for appointments." Notice

that this is *a very basic set of cues for practicing the "calendar-checking" process*:
1) alarm clock [a behavioral cue: startle reflex];
2) query about today's activities [a semantic cue];
3) query about whether there are specific appointments today [a more specific semantic cue]; and
4) question about checking the calendar or daybook [variable cue: visual, tactile, or imitative, depending upon the gesture(s) of the caregiver, e.g., pointing, reaching for the calendar, handing the calendar to the other person].

The foregoing cues are related to the calendar-checking process, and therefore, might be practiced every day. That cue hierarchy is not specifically designed for cueing memory about a haircut and has no semantic ties to haircuts, per se. *Instead it cues a basic procedure (of calendar-checking).* Items 1 – 4 (above) can help a person learn a process which might lead him/her to attend better to a day's demands and activities by fostering the activity that will lead him/her to find out about daily appointments. Over time, performance of the procedure can improve, and there is research to suggest that someone with AD can learn a procedure to support his/her memory (Knopman & Nissen, 1987; Poe & Seifert, 1997; Seifert & Baker, 1998).[1]

Some interventions can improve memory while enhancing ADL's and IADL's (respectively, activities of daily living, like obligatory bathing and locomotion; instrumental activities of daily living, such as using the phone or cooking; Gitlin et al., 2006). *Practicing skills* like bed-to-chair or chair-to-standing transfer might benefit individuals and their caregivers, too. The caregiver can build a procedural hierarchy with cues for the physical movements that are ordered in a sequence from "start" to "finish". Like the cues for calendar-checking (above), these can cue a *process*, rather than a specific fact/event (like remembering a haircut on a given day). As an example, build a procedural hierarchy for rising from a bed (supine position) in which the PwD is asked to complete a specific series of steps every time s/he arises (e.g., open eyes, fixate a landmark on the ceiling, look to the preferred side, fixate on that side's bed rail, grip that bed rail, pull one's torso up, shimmy hips sideways, dangle one's feet over the side of the bed, grasp one's walker with both hands, etc.). Persons with dementia can practice the steps many times as "exercise" (and over many days), so that getting up in such a way becomes an automatized habit, which depends little on conscious recollection for its successful completion (for intervention strategies, see Gitlin et al.; Vu, Weintraub, Rubenstein, 2005).

Another approach to building a cue hierarchy is to provide specific cues related to the actual content of the memory to be retrieved (e.g., a haircut). The alarm clock awakens the individual, and we ask what s/he has to do today. The cues that follow are all semantically related to getting a haircut. Upon failing to cue the person with this query, we then proceed to toss our hair or brush our fingers through our own hair (an admittedly subtle cue). Lacking success with that probe, we might ask whether s/he will bathe and dress—noting that his/her hair looks a bit long. For some folks, that does the trick: with a mention of hair length being enough for correct recall about the morning's hair appointment. For someone with more severe memory difficulties, we might have to prompt with, "I think your haircut is coming up soon. Let's check the calendar to find out whether it is today." Notice that the specificity of the cues increases as we move down the cue hierarchy from general to more direct, specific cues. The semantic cue hierarchy can include words, visual cues, and gestures *that are related to the meaning* of the goal response (e.g., hair, hair length, personal hygiene).

If you're confused about how to categorize cue types, remember that any cue which relates to meaning [an item's category (like "shirt" as a type of "clothing") or meaning (what it *is*: with a haircut being related to one's head, his/her appearance, beauty salons/barbershops)] is fundamentally "semantic". Cues are also labeled according to their modalities (e.g., sight, sound, touch, smell; like the potent aroma of a favorite shampoo being directly related to hygiene and one's hair). Thus, when I ask an elder to "look at the calendar" in order to probe his/her memory for a hair appointment, the cue is verbal (and perhaps gestural and visual—if I point to the calendar on the wall). However, the cue to calendar-check is not semantically related to haircut, because the directive to calendar-look contains no information about hair or a haircut.

It is important that research recommends to use *either* spaced-retrieval practice *or* a cue hierarchy, *but not both at once* (Bourgeois et al., 2003). *Cue hierarchies allow retrieval failures.* Errors are permitted and the task provides successively bigger clues for jogging memory. *Alternatively, spaced-retrieval's benefit depends directly on supporting successful memory retrieval (i.e., correct answers) at every attempt to retrieve.* It's one of the big reasons that spaced-retrieval tasks for forgetful individuals begin with very short intervals [e.g., by directing, "This is your personal calendar," and then after 20 seconds asking, "What is this?" while showing the forgetful individual the calendar]. Because its focus is different, the cue hierarchy can decrease the effectiveness of a spaced-retrieval schedule, if the two techniques are co-mingled (Bourgeois et al.). An incorrect answer (perhaps from an insufficient cue) would cause the teacher to drop back to a shorter interval (in the spaced-retrieval schema) before probing again, thereby interfering with achievement of recall at a longer spaced-retrieval interval.

Cognition and Performing Skilled Tasks, Like Driving

With respect to basic skills, there do seem to be some limits imposed by an aging body. Elders perform more slowly than younger adults on speeded tasks that require perceptual skills or psychomotor coordination (Whitbourne, 2001; Rowe & Kahn, 1998; Schaie & Willis, 2002). Elders also score lower on tests of physical strength (Whitbourne; DiGiovanna, 1994; Kirasic, 2004). However, with aging there also seems to be an emphasis on accuracy (e.g., Schaie, 1996). The proverb, "Haste makes waste," (Publius Syrus, 42 B.C./2000, Maxim 557) takes on added significance as many elders begin to evaluate performance differently than younger adults (as in Schaie & Willis, pp. 347-351; Berk, 2001, pp. 508-509). In a see-saw of what cognitive psychologists call the "speed-accuracy tradeoff", elders seem to have more anxiety about errors, while younger adults are generally more risk-taking (a fact which might be related to different emotional self-regulation in elders; Williams, 2006; Mather & Carstensen, 2005). Ruth and Birren (1985) discussed the ramifications of elders' error reluctance in problem solving tasks. An older adult might be less willing to accept performance with *any* errors. As a result, s/he might take steps to reduce mistakes: by being less creative and conforming more to social conventions (Ruth & Birren), or by slowing down considerably on tasks that require quick responses (i.e., in order to check for accuracy; Berk, 2001).

It's very interesting to note that an increased emphasis on accuracy can pay off for older adults. Data on automobile accidents indicate that there is relative sameness in the number of insurance claims for vehicle accidents (reported per 1,000 insured vehicles) among drivers aged 25 to 70 years. It is among drivers younger than 25 and over 70 that claims occur more often (with inexperience for those under 25, and slowing reflexes and changed senses in those over 70 most likely playing key roles; Insurance Institute for Highway Safety, 2003; Garzia & Trick, 1992).

About Aging and Intelligence

With respect to solving the problems of everyday existence (like "finding a place to live" or balancing one's checkbook; see Schaie, 1996, for a description of some of this research), the ability to confront a novel problem and solve it is part of what scientists call "fluid intelligence". For tasks that draw upon previous experiences (such as solving a problem via the facts and skills you've learned), the abilities are part of "crystallized intelligence" (Horn & Cattell, 1966). It has been reported in several studies (and across different countries) that average fluid intelligence seems to decline with age. Conversely, crystallized intelligence seems to increase with age (but perhaps not beyond age 74; Schaie & Willis, 2002).

With respect to knowledge of language usage, history, and cultural changes, this crystallized intelligence can show up as wisdom, and it can be evident in the abilities of older adults to out-perform younger adults (as in games like Trivial Pursuit[TM]— provided the emphasis is *not on the speed of responding*). Some writers emphasize "wisdom" over "intelligence" (Bolt, 2004). An individual who possesses wisdom might be practical, creative, and analytical in ways that transcend the traditional assessment of intelligence (as in traditional measurement such as IQ tests; Sternberg, 1997). Emerging literature in positive psychology slates wisdom as one of the six most desirable human traits (see Peterson & Seligman, 2004).

About the caveat that an aging advantage in crystallized intelligence might disappear among the very old (in octogenarians and beyond), it could be affected by a phenomenon known as "terminal drop" (Kleemeier; Davies; both as cited by Riegel & Riegel, 1972). Although it is unclear why, it has been reported that many older people experience a marked cognitive decline in the year(s) just before death (among those who die in old age due to health-related causes rather than accidental/unexpected deaths; Bosworth, Schaie, Willis, & Siegler, 1999; Fillit & Butler, 1997). In their research, Bosworth et al. (1999) reported that time-to-death (the elapsed time between the most recent intelligence test and one's death) was a small, but significant aspect [accounting for about 1 to 3% of the (unique) variance in a regression model] of poor performance on tests of intelligence in the Seattle Longitudinal Study. That is, for individuals who participated in the study, a shorter time to death was paired with a lower test score, compared to other participants. Other factors, such as education and age seem to interact with time-to-death, though, as predictors of a single individual's decline in test scores over repeated measures. In sum, studies that attempt to model cognitive decline in old age should consider time-to-death as just one of many variables that might predict cognitive function (Bosworth et al.). Unfortunately, such a factor is necessarily "post-hoc", because we cannot know a person's time-to-death until *after* s/he has died. It's only then that we can go back and apply it as a factor in a model to account for cognitive performance and decline.

Common sense can prevail as we attempt to understand the phenomenon of terminal drop. After all, among the very old, illnesses that lead to death can influence functioning of major body systems and individual organs. As those systems cease to function properly, they can diminish a person's overall level of cognitive functioning, because: 1) the individual does not feel physically well enough to perform with acumen on tests or cognitive tasks, and 2) vital physiological processes which affect cognition (like circulation of oxygen and nutrients in the blood) can be compromised (Bosworth et al., 1999). In the section that follows, I will describe one application in cognition that derives from my own study of reading among individuals with moderate-to-severe dementia of the Alzheimer-type.

Application: Without Words

Ruth Abraham (2005) wrote an insightful book about the use of art therapy to help individuals with dementia to communicate their thoughts and emotions. More generally, many older adults suffer from illnesses or injuries (e.g., stroke, Alzheimer's disease, Parkinson's disease) that interfere with their abilities to express emotion or communicate. I've thought of the poem, *Burnt Norton*, written by T.S. Eliot, and Abraham has aptly reiterated select lines from it in the introduction to her book: "Words strain, Crack and sometimes break..." (Eliot, 1935/1991, p. 180; see also, Abraham, p. 1). Reality of life—for individuals of any age—is that communication isn't always easy. Sometimes the basic mechanisms of speaking, listening, reading, and writing are disrupted. In two decades of work in gerontology, I have seen many different cases, and the reasons for communication difficulties have varied. In my specific experiences with individuals who have Alzheimer-type dementia, reading is a basic skill that remains intact long into the course of their illness (e.g., Newroth & Newroth, 1980; as reprinted in Janicki & Dalton, 1999, Appendix 2). Among enduring skills, reading can be used to communicate with individuals with dementia and to help them remain active participants in their environment.[2]

For seven years, I assisted two groups of residents at two different long-term care facilities in the Midwest. I have directed specific, timed (1-2 hours) activities for them once or twice a week. At times, these residents have been participants in research studies to test intervention strategies for Alzheimer-type dementia ["DAT": the cognitive problems that accompany Alzheimer's disease; as I mentioned previously]. When I wasn't running a specific research study, I provided my services as a volunteer to direct assorted games and activities—some of which actually originated in my research (e.g., art activities, trivia games, games with prizes, card games). Most of these activities utilize simple instructions and fairly simple procedures. A game might consist of three or four sub-components, such as: 1) reading a word or phrase that has been block-printed on an index card, 2) following the instructions on the card (e.g., "Open the blue drawer."), and 3) assessing the consequence to establish a state of "winning" or "losing" the game (like finding a small chocolate bar in the blue drawer when all other drawers in a small cabinet are empty; see Footnote 3, below).

As I mentioned before, a common element of many of the games and activities I have innovated is simply "the index card". I use ruled index cards of 4 in X 6 in (10.16 cm X 15.24 cm) or 3 in X 5 in (7.5 cm X 12.5 cm) index cards with block print (black ink from a permanent marker on a white, ruled card). Generally, the print should be on the ruled side of the card, and the other side should be left completely blank. If the lines on the cards seem to be especially problematic for an individual's success in reading, it is easy enough to duplicate cards on un-ruled cardstock. The most common feature of words on the cards is to have printed (not script or cursive) words with letters in lower case. Line thickness for letters is 2-3 mm (.12 - .18 in), and whole letters are approximately 1 cm X 1 cm, each. Again, the letters are usually lower case, except in the rare instances when a proper noun is used or when the text is a complete sentence—both of which would begin with a capital letter.

With respect to verbal instructions on tasks that utilize index cards, I spend very little time explaining an activity. Generally, I'll provide a couple of sentences aloud to give the gist of the task (e.g., "This is a trivia game. I'll ask the questions, and you try to call out the answers."). Because Alzheimer's disease and related dementia influence a person's ability to hold information in conscious awareness, it is not a good idea to give detailed or lengthy instructions. They can overwhelm a person with AD, and are not likely to be well understood—especially when someone's disease has progressed beyond the early stages. The most likely response to a long set of verbal instructions is: "What? I've never been here before," or "What should I do?" or "I don't know what this is." Feeling confused or overwhelmed by several sentences of verbal instruction, a person with dementia might try to leave the session, might become disruptive and abusive, or might use repetitive questioning (e.g., "What am I supposed to do here?").

Many of the activities I've designed share common procedures. When a new "turn" begins, I shuffle approximately six index cards and fan them out in my hands, so that the printed sides are face down (with the blank sides face up). Then, I lean toward a particular individual and say, "Pick a card—any card." I utter the sentence like a magician who is beginning a card trick. It's such a familiar expression (and they hear me say it so often) that participants often repeat it with me. This provides testimony to benefits of spaced rehearsal (as described previously; Camp et al., 1996). Participants become so familiar with the technique that the deck of cards fanned out in front of them becomes a cue for saying, "Pick a card—any card," with a motion to reach out and choose one.

When a player reaches out to take a card, I instruct, "What does the card say?...Please, read it." The latter sentence is key: a directive to read. Individuals with Alzheimer's disease often develop a tendency to respond to any question with "no" (probably because they do not fully comprehend the questions and might be leery of making an error; Mace & Rabins, 1991). When I prompt with, "Read the card," a person with AD will often read it aloud, because reading is automatic—i.e., a very common and "over-learned" skill. In fact, reading stays long into the course of this disease, and it is often the case that individuals who have advanced far into Alzheimer's disease can read aloud quite well (e.g., Hamdy, Turnbull, Edwards, & Lancaster, 1998).

Depending upon the specific game or activity, reading an index card might lead to one of several different outcomes. In a trivia game, the participant might select a card that directs us to "Go to the green envelope" or "Choose red". I proceed to pull a trivia card from the specified envelope (e.g., the red one). Generally, I set up this type of game on a large bulletin board or poster board. In the trivia game, when I pull the trivia question from the specified slot or envelope and read it, participants then try to give an answer. If the group is arranged in a semi-circle, individuals can call out their responses and need not wait to be called on. A correct response might win the respondent a prize, or it might lead to the distribution of a "celebratory prize" (like a piece of chocolate for everyone in the group in celebration that someone has come up with a correct response).[3]

For caregivers or staff who direct activities, it's very important to know the needs of the group. Some strong personalities or individuals with moderate-to-severe cognitive impairment might be less patient when only one person wins; They might all expect to receive a prize. Gauge 1) whether individual winners can be awarded solo prizes, or 2) whether prizes for all players are more appropriate. Do this by knowing the personalities, interpersonal issues, and levels of functioning among your activity group's participants. In Appendix B of this volume, I have given step-by-step examples for several activities for groups for persons with DAT. Changing tasks just slightly can make them feasible for groups of individuals without dementia, too. Elders who have no cognitive impairments are generally more tolerant of activities that award a single winner with a prize, and they are generally more tolerant of fast-paced games and tasks. But beware! It is absolutely critical to understand the personalities involved, because one group can be entirely different than another. This is a lesson not lost on teachers (my teaching experience being over fifteen years, now), who often remark that a single class can have its own "personality", which is also different than the mere sum of its member-student personalities. I believe the same is true of activity groups! [4]

Application: With Words on
Index Cards

Activities with index cards that use the card-selection paradigm can actually yield valuable information about participants' alertness, orientation-to-task, and reading skills. I have archival data about reading skills that were gleaned from games like the trivia task described above. I have observed a general trend: that participants who have moderate-to-severe dementia of the Alzheimer-type are more likely to read an index card successfully on one occasion, if they have successfully read aloud one or two words from an index card in the two weeks previously. A participant's second failure reading aloud is a predictor of continued decline in reading performance (except in cases of acute illness/injury that might diminish reading performance temporarily and be followed by recovery). For nineteen individuals (aged 74 – 100) with DAT or related dementia whose reading performance is archived over a nine-month interval, I have assessed successful phrase, whole-word, and letter-by-letter reading. The following is my scoring system:

4 (Highest Possible Score) = with the participant reading all index cards correctly on each of his/her turns in the game (e.g., single cards with phrases like, "Choose red", "Select blue", "Pick green", "Move 1 level");

3 = with the participant making no more than one pronunciation error per index card, and with all errors in pronunciation being phonetically close to the target word (e.g., saying "bridge" for the target "bride" or "brew" for the target "bear");

2 = with the participant generally naming single letters or digits correctly but not reading whole words; infrequent (once per game) whole-word reading [almost exclusively of color names, like "blue" or "red" (which are high-frequency, over-learned words) without additional whole-word reading];

1= with the participant occasionally looking at the index card and naming a letter or digit on it; and with occasional mimicry after the activity leader/researcher has read the index card for him/her; and

0 = with no correct identifications or imitated reading of whole words and no orientation to the index card (no looking).

Unfortunately, I have not tested reading effects for individuals with pAD against those for age-matched controls. However, my limited, longitudinal data (i.e., for individuals who read index cards once per week in the trivia games; Seifert, 2006) can be interpreted as partial evidence of a beneficial effect of practice: to maintain reading during decline from dementia.[5] Participants with moderate-to-severe DAT exhibit fluctuations in reading performance over time, but frequent (i.e., weekly or biweekly) practice can help to counteract the effects of decline from dementia. Many participants (even with severe dementia) can exhibit sustained whole-word reading with weekly (or biweekly) practice.

Interestingly, too, if an individual with probable Alzheimer's disease has failed to read an index card aloud and correctly during each of two previous consecutive weeks, then it is unlikely that s/he will read such a card correctly during the current week's session of trivia (or a similar game involving index cards and card selection, as specified in the previous paragraphs). The most striking phenomenon in the data I've analyzed is that failure to exhibit whole-word reading at two consecutive sessions (generally 1-2 weeks apart, depending on the participant and his/her attendance at activity sessions) is a strong predictor of future failures.

Among 19 participants, 100% of those who failed to read whole words on two consecutive occasions (N = 5) also failed at later attempts to read whole words. Indeed, in otherwise physically healthy individuals with DAT or related dementia, the decline of whole-word reading to letter-by-letter reading seemed to portend an overall decline in reading performance (and cognitive function; Seifert, 2006).

The idea that practice might help maintain reading longer in dementia is consistent with other researchers' conclusions that older adults might experience important benefits from practice on cognitive tests. Rabbitt et al. (2001) have also reported that there are pronounced individual differences—something that I have observed in my research, as well. Overall, elder activities that provide opportunities for practice are desirable—as long as the practiced tasks are useful for maintaining function and are enjoyable for the individual. Not surprisingly, practice can play a role in social habits, as well. In additional sections of this book, I discuss the importance of nurturing social bonds and facilitating emotional well-being [See "Application: Individualized Needs for Affiliation and Involvement" (Chapter 2); also Chapter 3; and Chapter 5 (on emotion)]. In the next chapter, I describe an approach to emotional well-being which includes a strong emphasis on "practicing" positive coping. Here, again, we will see that practice is critical. It can help a person maintain skills for reacting to emotional events and stimuli in constructive ways.

5

Emotions and the Later Years

In Chapter 3 of this volume, I described a little bit about Ekman's (e.g., 1994, 2003) work on human facial expressions. *Although there is debate about whether some expressions of emotion on the human face are innate (Campos et al., 2004), there does seem to be general agreement that we use the facial expressions of other people to predict their behavior.* As I described before, a natural "over-smile" is an erroneous indicator of negative emotion. When a person's eyebrows are naturally arched and dark, an observer might misinterpret them as an indicator of surprise, fear, or even disapproval. Ekman's work and research by others indicate that two of most confusable facial expressions across human cultures correspond to fear and surprise (Ekman, 2003, p.11). Because a raised or arched set of eyebrows contributes to the "confusability", it stands to reason that my naturally high, arched eyebrows can contribute to others' misunderstandings about the emotion displayed on my face. If we add to this equation that I frequently work with individuals who are experiencing cognitive impairments (usually due to Alzheimer-type dementia), then we have a formula for disaster—in which I frighten people by appearing to be personally frightened or surprised. As I said in Chapter 3, I try to prevent this "alarming effect" by toning down my expressions. Intentionally, I try to furrow (lower) my brow a bit (which on me—merely looks like an average brow line). In that way, I don't take on the look of a raised brow, and as a result, I avoid giving an impression of surprise or disapproval.

Beyond the issue of avoiding the appearance of a negative facial expression for its own sake, there is an issue about stealing another person's attention. Eastwood, Smilek, and Merikle (2003) have demonstrated that adults are more distracted (from a simple counting task) by facial expressions that show negative emotion than they are by positive or neutral expressions. Apparently, negative facial expressions distract onlookers to the "global level" of the face— thereby removing attention from a person's primary task and from the specific details of the face being viewed. Interestingly, it is possible to conceive of this phenomenon as adaptive. If a negative facial expression—displayed by another person—signals a threat or something to be feared, then it is adaptive to have one's attention pulled to that negative facial expression, to the possible threat, and away from what s/he was doing. A person can then assess the potential threat and act, if necessary. Unfortunately, my "over-smile" (which *is* a smile and is not meant to be threatening—despite my arched brow) adds a detrimental distraction. It makes sense for me, then, to try to tone down what might appear to be a negative facial expression, so that I do not unnecessarily distract participants with DAT from the tasks on which they are focused. [1]

All this talk about my own facial features and expressions is not intended to be an ego-rant: "Oh, my face! My face! I just want to talk about my face all day long!" Instead, my goal is to emphasize the critical importance of **monitoring your own facial expressions** *and expressions of emotion when you are interacting with other people.* What information do you wish to convey? How do you wish to affect people around you? *Emotions are quickly formed, but they can linger as moods and as lasting impressions of others—formed, on some occasions, via interpretation of their facial expressions* (see Rosenberg, 1998).[2] What lasting impression do you intend to make on people around you? If you are a caregiver, how do your facial expressions communicate negative or positive emotions to those for whom you provide care? If you are caring for someone with dementia, it is important to realize that your facial expressions can have a profound influence on the emotions of someone for whom you care-give. With reduced abilities to manage and regulate their own emotions, people with dementia depend on others to help them maintain positive moods: a very important issue for quality-of-life (abbreviated QOL; Lawton, 1997)!

Application: Practicing Pleasing Faces

I use a very simple technique to find positive facial expressions. First, I stand in front of a well-lighted mirror and do "facial calisthenics". This is a 60-second routine: Smile, frown, yawn, and then repeat. Spend about ten seconds on each expression. If you have time, include an "angry face". Afterward, return to your smile. Try several versions of it. How does your smile look with a closed mouth? With an open mouth? Notice what your eyes and eyebrows do when you smile. Now, practice the smile that you like the most while thinking about something you like (such as your favorite flower, person, desserts, vacation spot, or color). Do you feel silly? Are you laughing at yourself yet? What happens to the smile? Do your eyes turn down at the corners while the corners of your mouth come up? Remember these aspects of the true smile, and practice moving your facial features to make that smile. This might help you to make a more genuine smile when you are "on the spot" with someone for whom you care-give. Most of all, practice smiling, because the mere act of putting on a smile can actually improve your current emotion (Adelmann & Zajonc, 1989)!

There is a complicated interplay between physiological drives, human motivation to satisfy those drives, patterns of neural (e.g., brain) activation that regulate drives and behaviors, and our experiences of those various states as pleasurable or painful (see Damasio, 1999, Ch. 2). Add social context and experience and it makes the 'equation of emotion' incredibly complicated. Shields (2005, p. 3) posited that "no less than the claim to authenticity and legitimacy of one's self-identity or group identity" is in jeopardy "in the everyday politics of emotion...." She also contended that determining the legitimacy of emotional expressions is in the hands of those who hold social power.[3] What's more, research indicates that learned patterns—which influence the display of one's emotions and the perceptions of others' emotions—may comprise "dialects" of the more universal emotional experience (Tomkins & McCarter, 1964; as discussed by Elfenbein & Ambady, 2003). There is an "in-group advantage" for evaluating facial expressions—which might depend, in part, on learning a specific culture's emotion dialect

(Elfenbein & Ambady). Broader contact with diverse cultures has been shown to improve evaluations of other groups' dialects of emotion expression (Elfenbein & Ambady).

Even a small group (like a nuclear family) can have its own dialect for expressing emotions. Shields (2005) pointed out that a person can break rules of appropriateness of emotion expression, management of emotion expression, and amount of emotion expressed. Violating the norms of the group can lead a person to be disliked by, ostracized by, or even expelled from the group.

It's important to study the expressions of emotion by those around us. Caregivers can commit to a study of the rules for expressing emotions that are communicated by others. I recall one of my great aunts—who was quietly sentimental but not prone to public displays of sentimentality. On a visit to her home, I received a beautiful gift from her. It is a doll I had played with during my childhood. I believe that this was an expression of her affection for me. She revealed her emotions and love through acts, like making a gift of a treasured object to me. However, she wasn't much for talking about emotions, and when I began to cry (being touched by the act of affection), she was embarrassed, blushed, and said, "Oh, goooood night!" I had heard her utter this exclamation before, i.e., on occasions when an emotion overwhelmed her. The spoken words helped to calm the tension of a highly emotional moment and aided the transition to another topic of discussion— signaling, if you will, the change to something less poignant. Here we find an example of the politics of emotion within a family with a simple verbalization serving as a signal that emotions run too high and as a transition to a topic or activity that is less emotional.

About Emotional Intelligence and Everyday Life

Emotions are not *just* facial expressions. In fact, some researchers take a view that humans can possess a measurable ability to interpret, process, understand, experience, and display emotions. In the 1930's, Robert Thorndike described some aspects of emotion in relation to social interaction; he called these skills "social intelligence" (as described by Grewal & Salovey, 2005). In the interim, others have suggested that performance on tests of intellect—and success in life—can be affected by personality and by factors other than cognitive abilities (e.g., Gardner, 1983). Gardner described two "frames of mind" that relate to: 1) a person's knowledge of self (intrapersonal intelligence), and 2) his/her knowledge about others and how to interact with them (interpersonal intelligence). Salovey, Mayer, Goldman, Turvey, and Palfai (1995) explained these emotional abilities and several others in terms of "emotional intelligence".[4] Essentially, these theorists posited the presence of specific skills for evaluating emotional content of situations and interactions, reacting to emotional events or material, and producing and interpreting one's own and others' reactions. With some elements of emotional intelligence being innate and other aspects being learned, it might be possible to measure an individual's "EQ" [termed this way to indicate the comparison with "IQ" —with the latter being an indicator of cognitive abilities (intelligence as traditionally defined); Goleman, 1995].

Salovey and Mayer (1990) conducted foundational work on emotional intelligence ("EI") that has led to formulation of a theory of EI and to the construction of tests to measure it. In follow-up work, Grewal and Salovey (2005, pp. 333-335) described four rudimentary aspects of EI: 1) "perceiving emotions"; 2) "using emotions" to aid thought and reasoning; 3) understanding basic emotions, their relationships, their representations, and transitions between them; and 4) "managing emotions" through such methods as mood regulation, persuasion, and impression management. Let's consider each of the four aspects and the implications for relationships with adults in late life.

According to Grewal and Salovey (2005, p. 333) "*perceiving emotions*, includes the abilities involved in identifying emotions in faces, voices, pictures, music and other stimuli." An individual with high EI related to perceiving emotions should be able to pinpoint emotions on the basis of evidence from such sources. This type of skill is critical for overall EI, because it marks the entry of emotion-based information into mental awareness. If a person misinterprets the emotions of others, it can lead to communication problems, hurt feelings, or even failed relationships. When it comes to the work of Ekman (cited above, e.g., 2003), universal rules for understanding emotional facial expressions are aptly conceived as part of the "perceiving emotions" domain of EI. It is very likely that humans inherit some skills associated with identifying emotions represented on the human face. Nevertheless, there are differences between individuals in their abilities to perform this basic function, and experience seems to influence perceiving-emotions-skill, too (see Pollak, 2000; as cited by Grewal & Salovey).

Just as people vary in abilities to perceive emotions, they differ in the extent to which aging senses impact this aspect of EI. Failing vision might interfere with an individual's otherwise excellent ability to discern the emotion represented on someone else's face.

Conversely, less acute vision might actually enhance perception of emotions by enhancing attention to the global level of representation of the face (i.e., because less acute vision would afford less information about local features). I conjecture here about this possibility, because research about interactions between aging senses and perceiving emotions is scant (see the chapter on aging senses, above, as well).

Another of the four dimensions of EI is revealed *when emotions aid reasoning, thinking, or problem solving* (Grewal & Salovey, 2005). Research indicates that depressed mood can negatively influence memory and problem solving. Conversely, positive mood might actually enhance thinking (e.g., by widening the field of a person's attention, by opening the range of considered options, and by broadening the range of possible actions/reactions; Fredrickson, 1998). Restated: a negative emotion might narrow one's focus, thought, or action, while a positive emotion might extend the scope of things to which one pays attention, the ideas s/he considers, and the possible actions s/he takes. Fredrickson (1998) argued that positive emotions (like joy, contentment, interest, and love) "broaden the individual's momentary thought-action repertoire, and in turn build the individual's enduring personal resources" (p. 307). Moreover, Isen and her colleagues have demonstrated that positive affective states (induced by viewing a humorous vignette on film) can enhance problem solving in a task that calls for an unusual solution (see Isen, Daubman, & Knowicki, 1987). Positive emotions can open up new horizons and provide new means of exploring them!

A third aspect of EI that was described by Salovey and his colleagues is related to *comprehending emotions and their relationships to one another* (Grewal & Salovey, 2005). This can include discerning one's own emotional state, having insights about emotional states of other people, and being able to understand how it is that emotions are related, e.g., that contentment and interest might lead to joy. Lyubomirsky, Sheldon, and Schkade (2005) reported that there are three variables with fundamental impacts on long-term happiness: a genetic predisposition to happiness, happiness-evoking life situations, and happiness-oriented activities. They also demonstrated a key link between happiness-oriented activities and one's long-term happiness. It stands to reason, according to the EI theory of Salovey and his colleagues (e.g., Grewal & Salovey), that someone who is high on the "understanding emotions" dimension should be able to recognize the influence of happiness-directed activities on his/her lingering happiness (also see Van Boven, 2005, for another study about the benefits of the experiential aspect of lasting happiness).

A final dimension of EI involves *managing personal emotions and those of others* (Grewal & Salovey, 2005). People who are high on this aspect of EI are skillful at regulating their own emotions and know how to impact the emotions of others. Grewal and Salovey pointed out that this "four-branch" theory of EI does not define the ethics of emotions (like whether someone who has high EI uses it to control others or to help others), and they have noted that the model does not predict whether someone will actually use EI skills to act in a manner that is socially desirable (see Salovey & Grewal, 2005). Ethical considerations about emotion regulation and using emotions to manage other people's impressions are clearly important, but they fall slightly beyond the scope of this chapter.

Critically important to the social and emotional lives of elders is their ability to understand and manage emotions, because it can greatly impact personal coping effectiveness and interpersonal relationships. For many of the elders with dementia with whom I have worked over the years, I've seen this aspect of EI to be, perhaps, the most diminished. Even in the early stages of Alzheimer's disease, individuals might show flat affect (no apparent emotion) and/or wildly erratic moods. They might have impaired abilities to identify their own emotions and those of others (e.g., Janicki & Dalton, 1999). If caregivers can provide cues for positive emotions and promote experiences that are likely to lead to lingering positive moods, then they have taken steps to rescue individuals with dementia from the mood-swings that are so much a part of their disease. On a more basic level—for all individuals—whether of normal cognitive abilities or with dementia and whether young or elderly—experiences that bring positive emotions can help to improve quality of life (Lawton, 1997). When we foster positive moods through our own smiles and attitudes, and when we do this in a way that shows *we care*, then we demonstrate that *we value others* and *we help them to feel valued.*

I was acquainted with a fine lady who loved to play the organ. It had been her great pleasure to play a church organ for many years, and she had memorized many favorite hymns. As her memories faded into cognitive decline, she derived enjoyment from time spent at an electric organ (which had registers, stops, two keyboards, and several pedals—very much like the church organs she had played in prior years). She played from memory and we sang along. It elevated her mood and the moods of those who sang as she played!

Emotion Regulation in Adulthood

With respect to aging and emotion regulation, Carstensen and her colleagues have posited a "socioemotional selectivity theory" (e.g., Lockenhoff & Carstensen, 2004; Kennedy, Mather, & Carstensen, 2004). Their view is that aging brings with it an increased focus on one's current emotional state. This change in focus with aging might be due, in part, to a perception that one has fewer years left to live (Lockenhoff & Carstensen). Some benefits of this changed focus among older adults might be better regulation of negative emotions and longer-lasting positive emotions. However, disadvantages can manifest in reduced orientation to life goals and in failure to focus on possible threats (i.e., because of focus on positive aspects).

Carstensen (see Bower, 1999) reported that older adults showed superiority in regulating emotions—to the benefit of positive ones—relative to younger adults. In a report about American adults from 18 to 84, Carstensen claimed that elders were more likely to report more positive emotions and fewer intense negative emotions. Using a "pager" to cue participants at random intervals, Carstensen observed that younger adults reported a wider range of emotions than their elders. As mentioned above, older participants reported less time in negative emotional states and longer-lasting positive emotional states. Some researchers have described the difference in negative emotions across adulthood as one related to autonomic response: that older adults experience less change in heart rate, skin conductance, respiration, and perspiration (all of which involve a reaction to stress by the autonomic nervous system; see Kunzmann & Gruhn, 2005). However, Kunzmann and Gruhn reported that older adults do experience autonomic reactions on par with younger adults when distressing stimuli are pertinent to their age. In a study of reactions to short films—about such things as dementia and the death of a loved one—they found similar physiological changes in younger and older adults. Moreover, the elders reported more intense negative emotions in response to film clips relevant to old age than did younger adults (Kunzmann & Gruhn). Shouldn't this be so, though? Stressors that are more *personally relevant* should evoke stronger emotional responses from people to whom they are relevant, right?

With respect to elder advantages in the regulation of emotions, Kunzmann, Kupperbusch, and Levenson (2005) have reported that older adults did not better regulate their negative emotions (compared to a group of younger adults) when watching short vignettes on film (involving medical procedures). Kunzmann et al.

framed their observations positively, though, stating that emotion regulation might be one skill that does not evidence age-related decrements in adulthood. While Lockenhoff and Carstensen (2004) have made a stronger case for age-superiority in regulation of emotions, Kunzmann and her colleagues are cautiously optimistic that older adults are at least as able to regulate their emotions as younger adults.

Research on emotion regulation is still in its infancy. A fundamental debate rages about whether a heterogeneous emotional response to a potential stressor impairs one's ability to solve a problem or to reason (Charles, 2005; Feldman Barrett & Gross, 2001) or whether it enhances and broadens one's perspective (Fredrickson, 1998; Kennedy et al., 2004; Lockenhoff & Carstensen, 2004). Because so much of the research to this point has investigated negative responses involving disgust and because so many studies have made cross-sectional comparisons, it is difficult to draw strong conclusions about aging effects. If further research shows a robust effect of emotion regulation with aging, then one benefit can be to tighten the research focus on this aspect of life in late adulthood.

Application: Rehearsing the Positives!

Armed with the knowledge that elders can regulate their emotions at least as well as younger adults, a caregiver can approach tasks and activities with attention to emotional cues and their impacts (about emotion regulation, see Lockenhoff & Carstensen, 2004). Even for aging individuals who have cognitive and/or physical impairments, activities can be designed to bring maximum payoff with respect to their benefits as emotion regulators and promoters. **An example would be a reminiscence activity.** For many elders— even those with dementia—memories of days long past still linger. Activities that cue reminiscing have shown great promise in promoting positive mood among elders (e.g., Zgola, 1990).

In their study of three hundred nuns, Kennedy et al. (2004) observed that emotion-focused reflection about one's responses to a previous survey led to more positive reports than did accuracy-oriented remembering. The oldest participants in their study seemed to be the most positive in their attributions of emotion to the remembered autobiographical events. For younger subjects (who seem to regulate negative emotional memories less well than their elder counterparts; Lockenhoff & Carstensen, 2004), being directed to reminisce while keeping an emotional focus did increase their attributions of positive emotions to memories (Kennedy et al.). Despite this improvement for younger participants, it did not appear to bring their memories up to the same degree of positivity as their elders' reflections (Figure 1; see Kennedy et al.).

Overall, if the goal is to evoke participants' positive emotions, reminiscence activities that focus on feelings about memories might be superior to those that stress "hammering out all the details." Careful selection of reminiscences of eustressing (positive) events (rather than distressing ones) should help, too! After all, many people don't want to think about the day of a parent's funeral, but would greatly benefit from reminiscing about good times they had with that parent. This is one type of activity that can benefit from information about participant histories.

I recall a simple activity we've conducted for several years at a local long-term care facility. Individuals sort through magazines to find pictures of a probed item. I might call out, "Ok, the first person to find a picture of a shoe wins this round!" A simpler directive is: "Please, find a picture of a shoe." This activity—which is designed for participants with mild cognitive impairments—prompts quick scans of magazine and catalog pages. As we search, I add reminiscence prompts, like, "Oh, these look like the shoes I wore to my senior prom! Oh, how handsome my date was!!!!" With smiles and giggles, some of our participants will talk about their experiences of high school dances and dating.

It's important to exercise discernment when inviting people to participate in specific activities. Very early in my use of the magazine treasure hunt in a "memory reflections" activity at one long-term care facility, we (i.e., myself in collaboration with the activity staff) decided that one resident would not be a good candidate for participation. Her teen years had been incredibly traumatic and included the experience of being sexually assaulted while she was on a date. Because of her mild cognitive impairment, she tended to focus on that trauma and its negative emotional components whenever someone brought up the topic of high school (and this is understandable!). Given the likelihood that reminiscing in this way would only cause her more emotional pain, we decided that a casual game of magazine treasure hunt with life review about high school would not be a fruitful endeavor for her. Taking special care in selection of reminiscence topics and building knowledge about participant histories are both imperative for successful cueing of positive emotions in the treasure hunt-reflections activity (Ch. 6, Bowlby, 1993; Bowlby Sifton, 2004).

For others who did participate in the group, biweekly reminiscence through magazine treasure hunt has been a productive way to rehearse memories that evoke positive emotions (like memories of one's first date, a husband's proposal of marriage, a person's first job, favorite holiday/meal). For normal functioning adults and for higher-functioning adults with dementia, I probe less often with a single topic, and I utilize different themes across sessions. In that way, I don't foster boredom through sameness in the activity.

Another method of reminiscing includes a "Decades" game (Seifert, 1998) in which participants listen to verbal descriptions of historical people and events. Then, they guess the decade into which the event or person fits best. Large posters and pictures can be used to prompt remembering, and they can fuel discussions about "What *we* were doing when this happened." More than ten years ago, I started using the Decades game as a probe for reminiscing among high functioning residents in long-term care. They enjoy describing the events of their lives, and we've had many conversations about people's careers, families, houses, and hobbies.

Slide shows and photos can provide another technique to spur reflection. If slides are becoming worn, they can be professionally transferred to CD's or other media for projection (using a computer and projector) or transferred to overhead transparencies (via a color copy machine) for overhead projection. I recall showing a series of vacation slides from across the USA and Canada. Pictures included many vacation spots and monuments that participants could recognize (Washington, D.C.; Yellowstone Park; St. Louis; New York City). These familiar landmarks prompted many happy discussions about family vacations and cherished events from childhood (including one lady's fabulous stories about summer days at a family cottage). Practice improves memory (Ebbinghaus, 1885/1964), and practicing positive emotions through reminiscence can improve a person's overall mood (Kennedy et al., 2004).

6

About the Spiritual Self

Pause. What are *you* doing? Does it *mean* something? Anything?

Questions about human significance are far-reaching. They transcend the moment and one life, ... reaching across centuries, conditions, languages, and customs.

When psychologist Gordon Allport (1950) wrote: "[I]t is the portion of personality that arises at the core of the life and is directed toward the infinite" (p. 161), he was describing the search for life's meaning through religion. Despite human interdependence for the survival of our species, Allport thought that the personal effort to have a "pact with the cosmos" (i.e., one's religiousness; p. 161) is necessarily and ultimately a solo flight. Many writer's of faith have described religiousness and spirituality in terms of a human soul's transcendence beyond culture and society to connect with God: with that connection being conceptualized as the ultimate communion, rather than a solitarian endeavor (e.g., MacKinlay, 2001). While some psychologists describe spiritual quests in terms of a "depth" approach—in which religion provides a route for expression of unconscious processes (e.g., Jung, 1933/1971; Rizzuto, 2006), there are others who promote an "attachment model"—describing spirituality relative to one's need for and manner of forming attachments to others and the world (Granqvist, 2006). Another group of scholars (neuroscientists) has gone so far as to relate religious experiences to interactions between neocortical processes that: 1) regulate cognitive dimensions of social life, and 2) coordinate emotion-based communications, reinforcement contingencies, and reaction planning (Azari, Missimer, & Seitz, 2005). Some neuroimages from cerebral blood flow (CBF; Azari et al.) analysis might provide support for the empiricist's argument against a depth approach. A neuroscience-based attachment model could use the filters of social and developmental psychology—with an eye toward brain processes that regulate social interactions and interpersonal attachments. However, a depth psychologist's rebuttal to this threat of reductionism might emphasize inaccessibility of the unconscious mind to scrutiny by neuroimaging and CBF analysis. In between the polar views of: 1) an unseen unconscious mind, and 2) a brain-built spirituality, there is room for many perspectives. Ultimately, the systems of neural activation, learning process, and unconscious phenomena that feed human spirituality seem highly interactive and complex.

Some psychologists describe the search for life's meaning as a quest for self-realization; we act on the world to achieve the optimal self (as in Maslow, 1970). Consistent with self-actualizing is a search for wisdom (either bestowed by God, or as some see it, divorced from any mythical, divine creator). Wisdom might involve an optimal balance between knowledge, virtue (behaviors that presumably benefit the common good), and positive outcomes [e.g., Erikson, as cited by Wulff, 1996; see Sternberg's (1998) discussion of "a balance theory of wisdom"]. Still others approach a discussion about religion, spirituality, and life's meaning from their own beliefs: like Freud, who thought that an intelligent and mature ego would eschew the idea of God. Further, Freud argued that religion is fantasy which feeds human neurosis and insecurity (see Wulff, pp. 50-52). Allport (1950) also approached a study of spirituality from his personal experiences. Beyond them, he maintained openness and a sense of the need for a scientist to remain neutral about the topics s/he studies. Unlike Freud's view, Allport's rests on the side of emphasizing faith and growth, rather than neurosis and pathology. Abraham Maslow (1966), whose faith tradition was Judaism, came to a psychology of religion with even more than Allport's openness to study sacred and mystical aspects of human life. The psychology of religion, like so many specialties in behavioral science, has room in it for diverse perspectives: keeping in mind that a psychological scientist's goal is to describe and explain the psychology of religion, rather than to decide whether someone's religion is "true" or not (on this point, see Paloutzian, 1996).

These days, in the U.S., the terms "religion" and "spirituality" are used somewhat interchangeably in the popular culture—with a sometimes more negative connotation on the former term (as in the dogma and "regimentation" of religion). Overall, "spirituality" seems to have a less negative meaning (such as awakening the spiritual self). Around the globe, and in different contexts, these terms take on different nuances, but the scientists' debate about nomenclature should not distract us from the larger question: about *seeking meaning in life*. What "meaning" *is* embodies much of the search and/or debate about religion and spirituality. People, through centuries, have argued about and endeavored to understand whether life has meaning beyond the mortal and the mundane. Is there anything "holy" or sacred? What is our relationship to the sacred? Why does it matter whether we are merely mortal or connected to the infinite? These are just some of the questions that people ask (Pargament, 1997).

Our search for life's meaning can be social and public, or it can be tremendously private. The former is "external religiousness". The latter is "internal religiousness" (Allport, 1950). Gordon Allport conceived of internal religiousness as generally more mature and integrative than external religiousness, but Batson, Schoenrade, and Ventis (1993; as cited by Wulff, 1996) have argued for a third manner of religious engagement called "quest" (an orientation that is more open and flexible). Debate about the existence of and measurement of these three religious styles has resulted in numerous studies and research articles. It seems clear, at this point in time, that the orientations are not aspects of one, underlying factor ("religiousness"). Whether they are three different dimensions of the spiritual self remains to be demonstrated (see Wulff).

Pargament (1999, p. 11) called religiousness, "a search for significance in ways related to the sacred." Whether the journey is more public or private might vary from person to person and from one interval to another in an individual's life.

In my review about aging, religion, and spirituality, I cited some authors' references to advancing age as a time of spiritual crescendo or as a time to define the meaning in life (Bianchi, 1982; McFadden, 1996; both cited by Seifert, 2002a). However, I argued that it is not age alone, but crisis also, that can bring a person eye-to-eye with the infinite (see Musgrave, 1997; Lindauer, 2003, pp. 4-10). As we age, we have more chance to confront crisis (noted, as well, by Wink & Dillon, 2002). Thus, life experiences might be the mediating conditions through which aging adults gather a sense of their own meaning in relation to sacred and holy things. Furthermore, having a sense of life's purpose might portend better, overall adjustment. Research on "spiritual well-being" indicates that discernment of purpose is one important predictor of positive outcomes following a life crisis (e.g., Fournier, 1998).

Prevailing models of spiritual development in adulthood emphasize growth and one's sense of well-being (Paloutzian & Ellison, 1979).[1] Conceptualizations of spiritual growth in adulthood vary from those that focus on late-life spirituality as an offshoot of negative or attenuated circumstances (e.g., illness, crisis, disability), to others that proclaim sagacity issuing from adult maturation (Frankl, 1984; Jung, 1930/1971). However, many studies have suffered from an inability to separate maturational processes from cohort effects. Cross-sectional studies have indicated age differences in spirituality without discerning whether they are manifestations of adult development or generation differences resulting from social, cultural, and historical circumstances (e.g., Fowler, 1981: whose theory indicates more mature faith among older adults; with supporting data in a study by Labouvie-Vief, DeVoe, & Bulka, 1989).

Moberg (1953) had studied personal adjustment and religion. He emphasized the positive roles of particular religious activities, because they can increase one's social support and thereby enhance a person's ability to come through a life crisis (such as ill-health) more successfully. Shand (1990) had shown stability in religiousness among 154 Amherst College students over 40 years. Those data indicate that moving into adulthood with a high level of faith commitment can foretell endurance of that faith during adulthood. Benson's (1992) cross-sectional study indicates something similar: stability, and sometimes growth in religiousness with aging, if a person has entered adulthood with high religiousness (see my review, Seifert, 2002a).

In their explanation of data from a longitudinal study of development in adulthood, Wink and Dillon (2002) reported a main effect for spirituality: with both males and females experiencing a significant boost in it from the late-middle years (ages 53 – 62) to the older years (68 – 79 years; ages in their Table 1, p.82). They also noted an interactive influence of "negative life events" (like significant illnesses, deaths, and relational conflicts) and "cognitive commitment" in early adulthood on participants' spirituality in later adulthood (later 60's to middle 70's). Cognitive commitment (measured via California Q-set; Block, 1978, as cited by Wink & Dillon) is generally associated with intellectual endeavors, independent thought, and a desire to find answers to questions through study and reflection. This interactive effect held for both genders, but intriguing was the absence of a *direct* effect of earlier negative life events on males' spirituality in late adulthood. [Only females in the study evidenced later life increases in spirituality as a *direct* effect of previous negative life events.] *Overall, for women and men, an early resolve to make sense out of life heavily influenced their ways of deciphering experiences. It modulated the effects of earlier distressing experiences on spirituality later in adulthood* (Wink & Dillon). One way to view those results is that people who were committed to understanding life in the early adult years grew spiritually through their interpretations of life crises.

Young adults' involvement in religious activities seems to predict later life religiosity (Shand, 1990; Benson, 1992; Wink & Dillon, 2002). Some early research fell short of determining whether this was due to a developmental trend or to a generational difference. Wink and Dillon's longitudinal evidence supports earlier involvement as one marker for later life quest and practice of one's spirituality.

About Meaning, Happiness, and Virtue

Across the literature, there are various ways of describing life's meaning. In a review of subjective well-being, Shmotkin (2005) highlighted the divided literature on happiness: with some writers emphasizing happiness as a state of more pleasure than pain and others describing its emergence from virtuous and significant undertakings. Happiness research indicates that some people do define life's meaning in terms of happiness. Interestingly, many people have a baseline level of personal happiness to which they generally return—even after catastrophic events (like being in a serious accident; Shmotkin) or after eustress-ing events (such as winning the lottery; Brickman, Coates, & Janoff-Bulman, 1978). Yes, it's true that even positive events can create stress, but instead of prompting distress, they can elicit "eustress".

What characteristics and behaviors (of ourselves and others) lead to positive outcomes in human life? What human strengths do we value?

In the literature on shared ideas of virtue, Dahlsgaard, Peterson, and Seligman (2005) surveyed eight theological and/or philosophical traditions (e.g., Confucian ideology, Hinduism, Christianity). Their goal was to identify a set of commonly valued human traits and behaviors. To do so, they surveyed prominent ideologies and identified six virtues: courage, justice, humanity, temperance, wisdom, and transcendence (see Dahlsgaard et al., p. 205; see, also, Peterson & Seligman, 2004). Their list of virtues is tantalizing. Even more intriguing is their claim that only "justice" and "humanity" are overtly stated across all of the ideologies they reviewed.[2]

Is there a set of virtues about which many people can agree, despite our widely disparate beliefs and faith traditions? If so, then can those common virtues provide a basis for more effective communication and action across cultures and traditions? Are these common virtues universal? Are they part of some pervasive, universal truth?

There are thousands of writers who have tackled the topics about life's meaning over hundreds of years. I hazard to guess that there are still more (i.e., billions of) people who have wrestled with and who do struggle with questions about their own significance.

Why are you here? What are you doing? Does it matter?

Why am I here? What am I doing? Does it matter?

Ultimately, your answers to questions like these will influence how you act and how you treat others. At the same time you are acting on the world, other people are doing so, too. Their views about meaning will affect their behaviors, and when you encounter someone whose view of life is very different from your own, tension might develop. Indeed, differences in perceptions about life's purposes have led to wars, crises, and catastrophes.

As it relates to people's perceptions of life's meaning, I've found a book chapter by Pargament and Ano (2004) to be especially insightful. They described comparative results from several studies of "psychoreligious interventions" (focused on one's spiritual self) and cognitive-behavioral techniques (which focus on changing thoughts and their related habits). For individuals coping with a potentially life-threatening illness (e.g., cancer), spiritual interventions were superior to cognitive ones in helping to maintain a client's well-being. Alternately, for individuals with a relatively benign, but disruptive illness (like fainting spells), it was more fruitful to apply cognitive-behavioral interventions than psychoreligious ones in order to lessen clients' anxiety. Among their suggestions, Pargament and Ano remarked that spiritual interventions (with a focus on "control, identity, relationships, and meaning"; p. 133) seem to be more effective for individuals who are suffering from a diminished or lost sense of control. The cognitive-behavioral interventions, on the other hand, seemed more effective for people who could receive fairly definitive help from a medical device (such as a cardiac pacemaker that would diminish or completely alleviate fainting; Cole & Pargament, 1999; Cole, Pargament, & Brownstein, 2000; with both reports as cited by Pargament & Ano).

Wink and Dillon (2002) and Pargament and Ano (2004) have reminded us about the importance of spirituality "in context". We define ourselves through life experiences, by connections to others, and through a belief that we have significance in relationship to something else (to God, to others, to physical health, to the universe, to time, to 3-dimensional space). To return to Allport's (1950) view, at the same time that he defined religion as essentially solitarian, I believe he described it as relational. The paradox is that he framed the problem as a singular search for personal meaning, but he set it in context: as a quest for one's *meaning in the universe.* Personal meaning is necessarily referent. As I mentioned in a previous chapter, and as throngs of people before me have observed: We don't exist in a vacuum. Even if I were alone and floating in outer space, then I would still have dependence on oxygen, water, and so on.

Your views about your own value and about the importance of other people have a tremendous impact on your daily life. If you take someone for granted, you might be communicating that you do not value him or her. If someone ignores you or berates you, s/he relays a sense of your worthlessness. In adult life, the processes whereby we review and reflect about our lives can lead us to a sense of "despair" or "integrity" about life's meaning (Erikson, as cited by Wulff, 1996). In his version of ego psychology, Erikson (1980) situated wisdom as a pinnacle achievement of old age. Establishing integrity, an aging adult displays wisdom, hope, and love (among the many manifestations of a mature ego about which Erikson wrote). Certainly, these aspects of a developing ego are widely valued human virtues (Dahlsgaard, Peterson, & Seligman, 2005).

You'll notice a specific theme in many of the "answers" to the puzzle of life's meaning: RELATIONSHIPS. Oodles of theologies, philosophies, and historical perspectives define a person's meaning in terms of an association with something or someone else. *People for whom we care or from whom we receive care exist in relationships with us, with others, and with the world.*

Application: Building Relationships through Reminiscence

One of the richest banks for building relationships is memory, and even elders who have dementia retain some aspects of memory long into the course of their disease. For elders who are well and for those who are not well, the value of reminiscing can be high. A small group of (6-15) people can create a social event, and a social event can be just the place for sharing stories about one's childhood, about one's career, about his/her children (and grandchildren, and *their* children), about one's life as a bachelor, about one's golfing trophies, about his/her travels, and about the triumphs of life! A simple story can set the stage for a short session (15-20 minutes) of discussion and reflection. I recall that a few years back, I heard a presentation by Camp and his colleagues about question-asking-reading (or "QAR"; 1998) for elders in long-term care. I'm uncertain whether that study (as reported at the 1998 Ohio Network of Educational Consultants in the field of Aging: "ONECA") has been published, but I thought it was very interesting. I'd read a previous report on QAR (Stevens,

King, & Camp, 1993), and I've adapted the task to small-group reminiscence in eldercare.

A simple story and a few questions (written in large, simple print on index cards) can provide a foundation for "themed reminiscing" (i.e., reflection that focuses on a specific theme). The activity session builds on a single topic, in order to foster remembering. Participants take part by listening, by reading questions from index cards, and by mentioning events/topics that relate to the story. It's generally a good idea to have pictures or objects available to cue discussion (e.g., a poster of a famous landmark for a conversation about that locale). However, be sure that props are large enough to be visible to group members and that they are safe (i.e., no sharp objects or small items that might go into the mouth of someone with AD, please). [In this volume, see Chapter 4 for index card specifications. See also, Appendix B.]

Themed Spiritual-Life Reminiscence

In the environment of long-term care (whether it's residential or daycare), religious and spiritual references might be few and occur seldom. Especially for individuals at secular facilities, the religious cues from their lives might be lost to boxes packed away for safekeeping. Without overt and explicit references to religious life, some elders can lose the sense of meaning they'd drawn from church services, religious books, and relics (like a cross on the wall or a framed verse). Increased interest in spiritual and religious supports has made its way into the eldercare literature (Leininger & McFarland, 2006; Nelson, 2002). I find Vance's (2004) chapter on 'spiritual activities' to be especially interesting, because he summarized basic activity strategies and stated specific ways to integrate religious cueing for several religious traditions (i.e., Buddhism, Christianity, Hinduism, Islam, and Judaism).

In an article about religious coping in dementia, Mindy Baker and I (Seifert & Baker, 2004; see also Chapter 2 of this book) discussed a few simple cases. Those illustrations give limited evidence for the benefit a person might experience when important treasures are maintained in his/her environment. Years ago, I worked with a gentleman who had severe dementia from probable Alzheimer's disease. He was extremely anxious. Hand wringing and echolalia (repeating the same sound or word again and again) were common behaviors. However, he responded to the Lord's Prayer and to the 23rd Psalm. When they were spoken, he would participate, and this seemed to calm him. These verses are relatively common "calming" ones for Christian individuals. For some people, music can serve a similar purpose: with a favorite hymn or song providing comfort when it is played on the stereo (or, even, performed live; see Goldsmith, 2001a; also, Goldsmith, 2001b). [For thematic reminiscence *for caregivers*, see Appendix C of this volume.]

To build a QAR session with spiritual/religious themes, start with poetry, a sacred text, a portion of scripture, or with a familiar Bible story. After you read it aloud to the group, give each participant an index card with a related question. For example, if the story is about Noah and the great flood, the beginning of the session can be as simple as: "I'm going to read the story of Noah, and then we can discuss it," (as uttered by the group leader). After a simple reading (5 – 10 minutes), start with one member of the group (and a circular configuration for participants' chairs works well here). Ask him/her to: "Please, read your index card." A sample question might be: "Why did Noah build a big boat?"

If group members are higher-functioning, then include more difficult questions, like, "Do you think that Noah was afraid during the great flood?" [It has more words, a more complicated sentence structure, and it relates to abstract ideas—not just to concrete objects.] Proceed around the circle, asking individuals to read their cards. As you go, ask participants about their views. Please, remember to repeat the question so that it stays in everyone's mind, and speak loudly enough so that everyone can hear you. The entire session can promote reflection. Don't be afraid to ask specific queries, such as: "Mr. XX, do you remember studying this story as a child? Did you wonder about all those people who laughed at Noah while he built the ark?"

Of course, this example will not be appropriate for every activity group and/or every facility. Although the session might work well for a group of individuals who are Christians and in long-term care at, say, a Methodist facility, it might not be appropriate at a facility where participants have many different backgrounds and do not share a common knowledge of Old Testament stories. For them, a different theme might work better.

Stories about children are entertaining for elders. They can reminisce about their own childhood, about their children, and about the joys of young life. Sometimes, I supplement story reading with visual aids: like objects that are described in the story, or pictures of hypothetical scenes. A picture of several children playing marbles can be enlarged and mounted on poster board. It can be propped at the front of the room (advisedly placed very near the activity leader, if the room is arranged like a classroom or lecture hall) and can be a focal point for attention. Let's say the group leader plans to read about a marble shooting competition. The poster can hold participants' attention and remind them about the topic of the story, both while it is being read and in the discussion session afterward.

A Story for Reminiscence: Marvin's Marbles [3]

As he walked to school, Marvin's only thought was about marbles. Which shooter would be best? Which marble would win the prize for him? He wanted to win the grand prize!

Several of the neighborhood children had entered the contest, and over the past two days, many of them had failed to qualify for the final round in the competition. It was Wednesday morning, and the grand finals would take place after school that day. Marvin would play against Jimmy Westhill and Newton Brown. He was very nervous.

As the school-day ended, the final bell rang, and children poured out onto the school's front lawn. A grassy area was roped off with bright yellow. Only two teachers, the school principal, and the three boys were allowed behind the ropes. The other children crowded around in front of them—staring at the three finalists and their marbles.

Miss Neno, the school's principal, called the boys, "Jimmy! Newton! Marvin! Please, come here. It's time to begin."

Each boy selected his best shooter. In turn, each tried, until finally...a tie!

"In the history of George Washington School, I've never seen it. It's a three-way-tie!" exclaimed Mr. Smithfield.

The teachers gathered under a big oak tree to make their decision about the marbles competition. Would they hold a tie-breaker?

"After much deliberation...we have decided...to hold a tie-breaker!" announced Miss Neno.

At once, the crowd of schoolchildren shouted. Children cheered and called the names of their favorite players.

"Hurray! Go, Marvin!" called some of them, and Marvin braced himself to shoot.

Jimmy and Newton both did well. Marvin would be the third to try, and as his shooter landed, the crowd went wild.

"Marvin! Marvin! Marvin!" they hollered.

For Marvin, it was a day to celebrate his trophy and it was a day of happy memories.

Questions for discussion cards:

(1) How many boys were in the final marbles competition?

(2) Do you recall the name of their school?

(3) Did you play marbles as a child?

(4) Was it a good idea for Miss Neno to break the tie?

(5) On what day of the week did the marbles competition happen?

(6) Where did they play marbles?

(7) Do you think children still play marbles today?

(8) Do you think Jimmy and Newton felt happy about losing the competition?

(9) What did Marvin win?

The foregoing sample story and questions are less oriented to specific religious lessons or perspectives than the QAR session about Noah. Instead, the latter is a story for reminiscing about childhood. Competitions are a common part of life. Spelling bees, baking contests, soapbox derbies, baseball games, beauty contests, and science fairs are part of many people's childhood experiences. To remember them through fiction (as in Marvin's story) is to create a platform for conversation, so that even the individual who never played marbles can hear about someone who did and identify with his/her emotions and experiences. You'll probably notice, too, that a story or poem can feed the human spirit, even if it isn't explicitly religious (see also, Appendix C).

It is true that—just as some people don't like to swim—some people will not enjoy a good short story and a time for discussing it. That's OK. If you work as a caregiver, activity staff member, nurse aid, or at another task in eldercare, you'll begin to notice whether a particular type of task is appropriate for the needs of a specific elder. You'll plan story-and-discussion groups with members in mind, and you'll begin to tailor topics to fit their joys!

7

About Creativity and Aging

Research and theory about human creativity are far too diverse for me to summarize them well in one book chapter. Instead, I'll focus on some key points about creativity, aging, and eldercare. Great scholars in the arts, philosophy, letters, and sciences have set themselves to the task of understanding and explaining this broad and fascinating topic (Cziksentmihalyi, 1990; for an overview, see Runco & Pritzker, 1999). At the forefront of research on creativity, psychologists have argued about the best approaches to measurement, including: 1) measuring creativity as a set of cognitive skills on a battery of tests (e.g., like tests of divergent thinking; McCrae, Arenberg, & Costa, 1987); 2) quantifying it as a function of creative products (e.g., an artist's recognized masterworks; Beard, 1874; Lehman, 1953); and 3) assessing creativity through biography and autobiography (e.g., such as books about a person or his/her personal interviews and notes; Galton, 1869; Lindauer, 2003). Overall, research on creativity during the last half of the twentieth century seemed to herald decline with age in adulthood (e.g., Lehman, 1966; Simonton, 1990). These conclusions have been widespread, despite the many narratives from creative elders and the many old-age masterworks that seem to indicate otherwise (Lindauer).

For years, there have been two main views of aging and creativity: *one of decline* [that derives mainly from cross-sectional research using creativity tests (e.g., Ruth & Birren, 1985) and creativity products (such as one's masterwork, if s/he is an artist or a writer; Lehman, 1953)], and *one of continuity* [that issues from longitudinal studies (like the Terman study of gifted individuals; see Holahan, Sears, & Cronbach, 1995; Torrance, 1977)]. Those who take the diminishment-with-aging view thrust forth tomes of quantitative research about creative productivity and tests of creativity as the evidence for creative decline—although the age of decline is hotly debated (for example, after age 30 v. between 30 and 50; Lehman; McCrae et al., 1987; Simonton, 1984; Root-Bernstein, 1999). Proponents of the creative-continuity view cite evidence (from longitudinal studies and psychobiographies) for stability—and sometimes growth—with aging (Galton, 1869; Lindauer, 2003).

The literature on human originality, flexibility, and productivity (all thought to contribute to creativity; Ruth & Birren, 1985) is complex and has a long history. With such prominent figures as Galton (1869) weighing in on the vote, it is already a long-lived debate. Lindauer (2003) indicated the tremendous range of possibilities for an elder: from despair in decline, to elation in personal growth with bursts of productivity. He pointed out the wide array of problems with creativity research: from the issue that elders are much less recently practiced at taking tests than younger adults, to the question about whether creative "products" and behaviors are accurate measures of a person's overall (mental) creativity. I recommend Lindauer's book to the reader who is serious about aging creativity research. It is an excellent starting place.

My purpose in this chapter is not to review all of the pro's and con's of definitions, paradigms, and approaches to the scientific study of creativity. Instead, I'd like to focus on what is arguably one of the most important products of that literature: accentuating a potential for creative endeavors in late-life (Torrance, 1977). For me, the question of heredity of creativity put forth so strongly by Galton (1869) is somewhat irrelevant. With a focus on applications to elder life and eldercare, *my key concern is whether I can foster creativity in individuals for whom I help to provide care.* My personal response to the question emphasizes adaptation. As so much of the literature on aging pinpoints: adaptation to life's challenges leads to generally better outcomes [e.g., in response to physical and health threats (Galton); in coping (Pargament, 1997)]. This leads me to the conclusion that a caregiver can try to identify ways of fostering adaptation to life's challenges through—among other things—personal creativity.

If I know about a person's interests, history, preferences, and limitations (e.g., from illness), then I can tap into her or his potential for creativity. Am I attending to a woman with gout who is in long-term care? Was she a ballroom dancer? Then, why not get some advice on technique as I play music and dance with various physically able residents (or staff). She might become the dance coach for the entire facility! Do I need to design activities for a group of community-dwelling ladies who are retired schoolteachers? Then why not use their expertise to get advice on my tutoring techniques for a child's evening math (or other) homework. I might devise a brief (10-minute) lesson on index cards or plain paper: illustrating my explanation of something like long division to a second- or third-grade child. When I present the lesson to these retired teachers, they can critique it and provide advice for its improvement. Or, if it's possible, give the ladies a chance to help a 7- or 8-year-old with her/his math lessons (e.g., running flashcards of multiplication with a child). These activities, designed with elders' personal strengths and limitations in mind, can give them some fantastic opportunities for creative problem solving!

Application: Art Expertise and Activities for Dementia Care

Current trends in dementia care emphasize person-centered orientation (Kitwood, 1993; 1997). With rediscovery of concern and regard for individual strengths and for a person's pre-morbid expertise, opportunities arise for improved dementia care. One area of exploration involves a study of individual expertise and the ways it changes over the course of Alzheimer's disease. The after-going includes information from my case study of an artist who experienced difficulties with prospective memory, planning, and retrieval of planned activities during execution of painting projects. The participant's history as an artist, and her diagnosis with probable Alzheimer's disease, informed my understanding about changes in her ability to make art and about her increasing need for memory cues in painting tasks. The case provides examples for planning and conducting painting (or craft) activities in person-centered dementia care.

Painting with Gina [1]

"The perspective is no good on these," Gina said as she handed the canvases to a staff member for disposal. This quiet and dignified woman, who had spent so many years of her adult life painting and teaching others to do so, was so completely dissatisfied with her own work that this was one of the last times she painted for us. Painting pictures—an activity which had brought so much joy to her and which had been so fruitful as a person-centered activity that we could perform with her—had ceased to bring her happiness.

I had met Gina shortly after her diagnosis with probable Alzheimer's disease. She was articulate, but shy, and her pre-morbid (before diagnosis with pAD) intelligence was probably above average (115-120 by our estimate and based on family reports and her biographical history). During the time I knew and worked with Gina her mental status declined from mild to moderate dementia (with MMSE = 21 initially; and MMSE = 17 at the termination of my observations). During that interval of just less than two years, Gina enjoyed sessions spent painting on canvas, on wood, and on paper. As her mental status declined, her enjoyment declined, but with more time and task re-structuring, I believe we could have observed the same success that I have documented in a previous case (Seifert, 2000).

Over many years of work with individuals who have Alzheimer-type dementia (DAT), I have observed a common phenomenon: that individuals will participate in activities for which they had achieved pre-morbid expertise only as long as their work continues to demonstrate that expertise. One older lady with moderate dementia completely gave up a traditional craft from her homeland in eastern Europe, because her skills had declined to a level that was unacceptable to her. She did, however, continue to enjoy conversations about the craft long after she'd abandoned practicing it!

Alternatively, a few of our participants have changed expectations to better fit their changing abilities. I recall the case of a gentleman who joked about his declining ability to complete woodworking projects. About them he said, "Hey, I'm a pretty old guy. I'm just glad to be able to do anything!"

My generalization that a person quits when s/he fails to perform at previously set, high standards is likely true for those who seem to have been very demanding of their own work pre-morbidly (and who perhaps, also, are "perfectionistic"; as indicated via family reports). In some cases, an assistant can provide cues to support performance, so that work continues to be of high caliber (e.g., Seifert, 2000). Memory and performance cues can perpetuate excellence and foster a sense of satisfaction in one's work (for sample cue hierarchies, see Chapter 5 of this book; see also, Bourgeois et al., 2003). Additionally, a caregiver can create an environment of acceptance in which s/he does not criticize the elders work, but instead, praises small victories in order to encourage and reinforce the elder's creative experience.

In prior studies, Mindy Baker and I observed that individuals who have mild-to-moderate DAT can benefit from structured activities which cue memory for facts and for procedures (Seifert & Baker, 1998; Seifert, 1998). We are not alone in reporting performance benefits from structured tasks and external cueing. Camp and his colleagues (e.g., Camp, et al., 1996) reported that activities which are designed to provide frequent external prompts are fruitful aids in dementia care. In the same year, Hutton, Sheppard, Rusted, and Ratner (1996) reported that structure in a "Subject Performed Task" (SPT; p. 113) can match encoding context with retrieval context in order to improve performance in a procedural learning task. Furthermore, salient cues at retrieval can prompt skilled performance (Bourgeois et al., 2003). The observations of Hutton et al. are particularly germane to art production tasks, because they suggest that motor routines, coordinated activities, and duplicated cues at encoding and retrieval are important keys to learning success among people with DAT. The finding is consistent with the general result that procedural skills can be trained and maintained in Alzheimer's disease—even when attempts to train declarative (fact-based) memories meet little success (Knopman & Nissen, 1987; Poe & Seifert, 1997). [2]

Applied to art activities (like painting and drawing), these techniques can be paired with age-appropriate and expertise-appropriate materials (for example, real canvas, paintbrushes, and artist-quality acrylic paints instead of elementary-school-quality art paper, glue, and construction paper). Both trained artists and novices who like to create arts-and-crafts can produce works that satisfy and gratify them. Hartan (1990) suggested that a key element in assisted art production is in "reading" the participant with dementia in order to provide collaborative support without "taking over" the project.

During my supervision of art activities with Gina, I observed that she became frustrated when she could no longer complete paintings on her own. Her ability to plan and execute artwork had diminished, because of her profound deficit in working memory. [Working memory is the mental "scratch-pad" that holds our current thoughts (Baddeley, 1997).] She would start to plan the layout of her work on canvas, and then in a moment—by a cruel act of disease—her plans would be gone from her conscious awareness. It was as if they had just disintegrated. Despite her difficulty with planning, her standards for excellence in her work remained high. Ideally, we would have continued to work with her in a "studio" atmosphere—i.e., as artists working side-by-side and commenting on each other's work. This technique was effective in a project I reported previously as I aided a woman to restore a family heirloom (Seifert, 2000). Each woman (i.e., Gina and the participant in the 2000-article) had high standards for her completed work, but each also needed assistance to plan parts of the task, to stay focused on short-term goals, and to be cued about the sub-routines she had planned.

When I work with individuals who are trained in visual art (or in a related field, like photography, ceramics, quilting), I adopt a strategy of peer-collaboration, and this seems to work well in cases involving mild-to-moderate dementia. In an environment of person-centered services, caregivers should consider the personality and history of the client/participant (Kitwood, 1997). For some individuals peer-collaboration might work best; for others, a mentoring role might be preferable (e.g., whereby s/he might "coach" the younger, less experienced artist). In still other situations, the client might prefer to be a "student" to a caregiver or staff member's "teacher" role. I have encountered cases of each type, and special diligence is needed in order to discover which role will suit the client who has dementia. Because the essential goal is to improve quality of life and well-being for the person with AD, it is vital that his/her comfort be assessed and monitored throughout the process of art production.

For Gina to act as mentor to me was a good fit for our relationship. She had enjoyed teaching others, and this skill for instruction could be brought into a structured environment. A tidy, uncluttered studio atmosphere with two tables or easels and a photo (in this scenario: a picture of a landscape) to use as a model for painting on a clean canvas: these materials provided the best way to promote satisfying art production. In this environment, Gina could "teach" me to produce better work. All the while, I could provide helpful questions that would cue her in her own work, like, "How would you start painting the trees? Should I begin by painting the foreground trees?" I might ask questions in order to cue her as she completed the canvas preparation, so that she might recall her next (planned) step, i.e., to begin roughing out foreground trees. At the same time, my questions were simple and non-threatening. In essence, I asked for assistance with my picture's composition, and she could offer helpful advice. The conversation served to maintain the current sub-goal in her conscious awareness.

After we had roughed out some trees and landscape features on our canvases, I might ask, "Now, how can I go about mixing a proper green for my pine trees? I want to fill them in with a darker green, right?" And she might respond by showing me how to do so. Importantly, I would continue to discuss these matters during the paint mixing, so that she would continue to be aware of the sub-task on which we were focused. My part of the conversation is vital as a reminder. Conversation helps the participant, because it reminds him/her of the current goal (e.g., to mix paint for pine trees, to select a brush that will help me paint leaves, to check my work against the model photo, and so on). Conversation cues memory. Thus, if it is on-topic and seeking advice, then "talk" can keep the participants on-task. If the conversation is unrelated to the task, it can be distracting and prompt a person to forget the current goals. Other distractions can come from a noisy, busy room that is prone to interruptions or from music and announcements on a loudspeaker.

In Lists 1 and 2 (that follow), I have provided a sample scenario of planning and carrying-out a painting task for an individual with mild-to-moderate DAT. This type of task might be appropriate for someone who is known to enjoy painting and who is also known to have some applicable expertise. The information in List 1 is intended to provide guidelines for planning the activity. List 2 provides sample dialog/actions for a painting (craft) session. No guarantee is made or implied about the applicability of these plans to an individual case. It is left to the qualified professional to decide about the appropriateness of these suggestions in their application to, or adaptation for, a specific client or patient.

List 1: Planning a Client-Centered Painting (Craft) Activity

Part I: Staff Preparation Phase

A. Explore the history of the participant (via family, friends, other caregivers).

1. Does the individual enjoy the planned activity?

2. Does s/he have special training or experience related to this activity?

3. Was the activity a hobby, profession, or both (something that might affect whether s/he views it as work, fun, or both)?

4. What types of work did s/he produce (e.g., portraits, photos, drawings, still life, landscapes, etc.)?

5. With what tools and in what mediums did s/he work (e.g., on canvas, on paper, with acrylic paints, with colored pencils...)?

6. In what type of environment did the participant engage in this activity (e.g., in a cluttered studio, in a classroom, in a neat and tidy office)?

7. Are there any client-conditions that might interfere with the success of the activity (like paralysis from stroke, physician or family objections)?

8. At what time of day is this client at his/her best?

9. Has the client been asked about his/her willingness to undertake the project?

B. Explore the options available for the activity in the current environment.

1. Are there any conditions in the current environment that might interfere with the success of this project (staff objections, lack of appropriate space, poor lighting, etc.)?

2. What might be the best location for this activity?

3. Can the activity be planned for a time of day and location that will lead to success (without noise, crowding, or interruptions)?

4. Are the needed materials available?

5. Can the room/location be set-up in a way that is favorable to client success?

6. Is an appropriate staff person/caregiver available to facilitate the activity?

Part II: Preparation for the Activity

A. The environment

1. Have all of the above (in Part I) questions been asked and answered?

2. Is all of the necessary paperwork (if long-term care, daycare, or clinic context) completed and approved?

3. Are the materials ready?

4. Is the room/location set-up?

5. Has the involved staff member/caregiver determined whether s/he will be peer, "pupil", or other?

B. The participant

1. Is the client well today?

2. Has s/he been invited to the activity before/while being taken into the room?

3. Is the staff member or caregiver providing enough verbal and non-verbal cues to support the client's performance without being directive? (See List 2)

4. Is the staff member or caregiver supporting a warm and friendly interaction that is appropriate to his/her knowledge of the client?

Part III: Undertaking the Activity

A. The environment

1. Have all of the above (in Parts I and II) questions been asked and answered?

2. Are the client and staff member/caregiver situated so that they can converse easily and make eye contact?

3. If the client is seated, then the staff member/caregiver should probably be seated as well.

4. Are all necessary materials within reach of the staff member?

B. The participant

1. Is the staff member/caregiver supporting the activity through conversation (List 2)?

2. Does the client appear to be comfortable?

List 2: A Sample Scenario of Conversation and Action in the Painting Task

Caregiver: "Hello, Mrs. XXX. How are you today?"

Client: "Fine, my dear. How are you?"

Caregiver: "Oh, I'm just fine. I've been enjoying the weather."

Client: "Me too."

Caregiver: "Mrs. XXX, I understand that you are interested in painting."

Client: "Yes, Honey. I used to paint."

Caregiver: "Oh, I love to paint. Tell me about your work!"

Client: "I worked with earth tones. I like to paint shapes and abstractions."

[Perhaps, as they walk together or as the caregiver pushes the client's wheelchair along the corridor.]

Caregiver: "Oh, this is so exciting for me, because I am interested in painting."

Client: "Really? What do you paint?"

Caregiver: "Oh, lots of things. In fact, I'm going to paint a picture right now. I'd love it if you will come with me. We could have some fun together!"

Client: "Really? ...Oh, I'm not sure."

Caregiver: "I sure would love it if you would paint a picture with me."

Client: "OK."

[As they enter the studio/activity center...]

Caregiver: "Do you like to work from a photo?" [Note that a proper history would have led the caregiver to have the room prepared just as the client might prefer— and with photos or still life arrangements already available.]

Client: "Well, Honey, I like to take a photo and make it my own."

Caregiver: "Will you give me some advice? I'd like to work with this canvas and build an abstracted set of shapes and textures from the photo."

Client: "OK" [Reaching out as the caregiver hands her a palette.]

Caregiver: "You mentioned earth tones. I have red, sand, and two shades of orange. I'll give us each some."

[As she says this, the caregiver dabs four blobs of paint onto her own palette and onto the palette of the client.]

Client: "Thank you. I like to arrange them toward the right."

Caregiver: "And do you prefer to have the colors arranged by the color wheel?"

Client: "No. Any order is OK."

[As she reaches for brushes...]

Caregiver: "I suppose we should prepare the canvas with background color. Which brush would be best for covering my entire canvas with the sandy color of paint?"

Client: [points to a particular brush]

Caregiver: [handing the same type of brush to the client] "Thank you. That seems like good advice, and I've pulled a brush out for you too. Will this brush work for you as you paint the background?"

Client: "It's perfect. Thank you."

[As they both start working on the canvas...]

Caregiver: "I believe this sandy-brown hue will be outstanding as a background color. What do you think about this color for the background—you know, behind the trees here?" [caregiver indicating areas by pointing or with the paintbrush]

One would proceed similarly and should follow the cues of the participant. Some individuals can maintain focus for 10-15 minutes of painting or artwork and tire easily, but others might have more stamina than the time available. Generally, I allocate no more than an hour or two daily for these types of activities, because I often find that space is at a premium—particularly in long-term care facilities. Moreover, while it is true that some individuals can maintain focus and paint for several hours, they may not be able to monitor their own levels of fatigue. This can lead to exhaustion, confusion, and disorientation from which an individual with dementia might not recover for several days. Overall, the **"Hour Rule"** is a good one: *with activity sessions for individuals with AD lasting no more than an hour.* This provides adequate stimulation for most individuals and can be followed by a brief interval of rest or by a snack. [My experience derives more from work with individuals who have late-onset type AD. For some individuals with early-onset type Alzheimer's, there may be better stamina, more energy, and a greater drive to stay at the task for more than an hour.]

I use the natural daily routine in order to schedule activities. For most individuals, the day begins with grooming and with breakfast. Then, there may be a naturally occurring interval of 1 – 3 hours before lunch. Many people are at their best during these hours just after breakfast. A study of a person's history can lead me to understand which individuals might benefit from an art activity during the morning hours. Alternatively, some persons are at their best in the afternoon, and for them the demands of an art activity are well-met after lunch. Finally, there are those folks who are "owls" (Guthrie, Ash, & Bendapudi, 1995). For any number of reasons (like years spent working a night-shift), these folks become bright-eyed after supper and may spend evening (and night) hours wandering. For them, a well-planned evening program can be the key that leads to a better period of sleep—leaving them with a sense of satisfaction and tiring them enough to prompt an interval of restful slumber!

Interestingly, Lynn Hasher and her colleagues (May, Hasher, & Foong, 2004) have recently reported that tasks requiring explicit retrieval of information (like taking a test about geography) are performed better during an individual's "peak" hours. However, tasks that rely more heavily on implicit (procedural) memory (like performing a dance routine, playing memorized piano music, or knitting) might not be dependent on a person's "peak" hours of the day/night for good performance (May, Hasher, & Foong). Whether these results will improve activity planning for individuals with AD remains to be determined. If the results are robust for the sub-population with AD, we might find ourselves planning more exercise, knitting, and painting activities during a person's "off-peak" hours.

Although my experiences and reflections can provide insights, they cannot be taken as set recommendations for specific cases that the reader might encounter. In dementia care planning, there no replacement for personal experience with a specific individual/client. **Depend on personal interactions, carefully collected historical information (e.g., from family, friends, other caregivers), and collaborating**

professionals to lead to excellent person-centered care for individuals with AD. Furthermore, stay alert to cues from clients that they are too tired, too distracted, or too ill to participate in a fruitful session. My memory of a client's words during a lung infection speaks volumes. She said, "Please, promise to work [paint] with me when I am done with coughing!" My reply: "You can count on it!" After she recovered, we enjoyed many more days of painting together.

Appendix A

A Hierarchy of Goals: Infusing Interventions into Individualized Care

[A View of Greenspan and Wieder's 'Integrated Intervention': Adapted to Eldercare by Seifert (to accompany this volume's Chapter 2)]

Top of the Intervention Hierarchy

5) person-centered interventions that are motivated by the specific history, preferences, and personality of the individual (e.g., reading aloud together with a retired pre-school teacher) AND support to transcend/transform *in context*, when/if possible (e.g., helping an artist with AD demonstrate brushwork to a small group of art students)

4) intervention strategies that promote independence and support one's current level of functioning, e.g., fostering independence by providing options (like meal times and food selections)

3) interactions to accentuate personal abilities and needs for sensing stimuli, interpreting incoming information, and planning actions, e.g., with a variety of activity choices—some active and some passive—like reading aloud v. listening to someone else read

2) structure for integrity in relationships, e.g., addressing individuals by name, in caring tones, and without "baby-talk"

1) support for medical/biological care and consideration of environment, e.g., through regular check-ups and attention to medications and physical changes, with care given to physical context *Bottom (level of entry) of Intervention Hierarchy (noting*

that, ideally, an elder regularly receives care across all levels of this hierarchy)

Appendix B

Three Activities with Index Cards

(to accompany Chapter 4)

A GENERAL NOTE: Having been around the block a few times with various facilities for eldercare and their activity staff members, let me say: You're right. That is, many activities and tasks I might recommend won't necessarily work swimmingly on the first try. This is true for multiple reasons, including their novelty to participants, your newness to the task and how it can be run, and trouble with participant selection. Over time, you'll adapt techniques to fit your needs and those of the elders for whom you provide care. In addition, I suggest what I like to call the **"Six Week Rule"**. Especially for older adults with dementia, *practice* can be one of the most critical components of success in activity management. In general, I find that **once-per-week for six weeks is a good test of an activity.** This usually provides the participants with enough practice that their familiarity (implicit, unconscious memories) with the task can counteract their failure to consciously remember it (explicit memories, which are often diminished in Alzheimer's disease and related disorders). Research indicates that older adults benefit from practice and that these benefits might, in fact, be greater than they are for younger adults (Rabbitt et al., 2001). About procedural skills and practice in Alzheimer's disease, see also Poe and Seifert (1997; while regarding Footnote 10, Chapter 2, this volume).

A CAUTIONARY NOTE: As a general principle, if you are working with individuals who have dementia, then be sure to supervise activities, and do not leave participants alone with activity materials. A moment of confusion can lead a person with dementia to attempt to eat something inedible (e.g., clay) or to use an object in a harmful way (e.g., attempting to use art scissors to open a cup of ice cream). Injuries are easier to prevent than to undo!

Activity 1: Top-of-the-Pyramid Game

Level of Skill: Mild-to-moderate Alzheimer's and related dementias

Materials: 3 rectangular, plastic nesting tubs that fit one-inside-the-next [e.g., (width X depth X height) 60 cm X 50 cm X 30 cm; 40 cm X 30 cm X 20 cm; 20 cm X 15 cm X 15 cm; with enough space to set a few knick-knacks on each level when the tubs are turned bottom-up and stacked like a pyramid]; 3-4 resin knick-knacks without small parts (e.g., a plastic basket of flowers approximately 6 cm X 6 cm X 10 cm, or a resin figurine—which does not look juvenile—of about the same size); and 1 set of 6-10 index cards (prepared as specified in Step 2, below).

"Playing" Time: Individual rounds (to reach the top) usually take only a few minutes. Play as many rounds as time allows, unless participants seem restless or bored. In my experience, 4-5 rounds are enough for most groups. After that, they've accumulated so many prizes that they become distracted by them. If the prize is a piece of candy (Footnote 2, Chapter 4), then limit the number of possible wins to snack allowance specifications at your facility. In general, I've found the limit to be 4 or fewer pieces of candy, but your facility's dietary guidelines might vary. [See Footnote 3, Chapter 4.]

Preparing Activity Materials:

1) **Be sure that the tubs stack bottom-sides-up and one-atop-the-next, like a pyramid.** There should be enough space at each level to set a few of the resin objects. Label each tub (upside-down, because tubs are stacked that way in the pyramid) with black

permanent marker. Be sure to use a bold enough marker and print-size large enough so that the labels can be seen by an older adult who is 6-8 ft away. Label the lowest tub in the pyramid with, "Level 1", and set all the knick-knacks on the table around the bottom tub. All knick-knacks start the game at Level 1, with the potential to move up. Turn the next-smallest tub upside-down and label it, "Level 2". Then, place it on top of the bottom tub. Finally, turn the smallest tub upside-down and label it, "Level 3". You might choose to denote the top, "TOP", by taping a labeled index card to a spare knick-knack or to a plain paper cup. The top need not be labeled, because the goal of the game (i.e., to get a knick-knack to move up to the top of the pyramid) is fairly obvious.

2) **Prepare index cards with simple instructions, like, "Move up 1 level," "Move down 1 level," "Move up 2 levels," "Move down 2 levels," and "Go back to Level 1."** In my game, we always stipulate that an item cannot be moved down below Level 1 or up above the top tier. That rule limits the pyramid movement to the playing (tub) surfaces. Be sure to follow instructions for printing index cards that were described in Chapter 4 of this volume. Also, I recommend that "1" on index cards should carry the features of an Arabic numeral (with top flourish to the left and a line segment footer), so that participants with moderate AD don't mistake it for "I" (which would lead to misreading a card as, "Move up I level" or "I move up a level").

Procedure:

1) Begin the game by setting up the pyramid and knick-knacks (with all knick-knacks starting on the table surface: Level 1).

2) Be sure the group of participants is assembled, and begin at random with a participant on either end—moving along the semi-circle as turns progress. For this game, the goal is to get one knick-knack all the way up to the top of the pyramid. Individuals

can play independently; or for groups who like team competition a group of 10 people can be set-up in 2-3 teams. If playing in teams, then each team can select a resin knick-knack to be their "game piece" in the pyramid. If the latter case, then a team member's selection of an index card will result in the movement of that team's knick-knack. If playing independently, then each player can select any one of the knick-knacks to move on a given turn, and they can choose to move a different one on each subsequent turn. This optimizes individual chances to win the game on a specific turn by getting any item to move up to the top.

3) Shuffle the index cards and fan them out. Hold them out, face down, and toward the person (or team) whose turn is current. Say, "Pick a card, any card." After the player selects a card, request, "What does the card say? Please, read it." For individuals with moderate dementia, some assistance might be required to help select the card. Then, hand it to the player with its orientation to that player. This will help the player notice that the stimulus is a card to be read. If the person fails to read the card (and this does happen, especially the first time the game is played, because the task is unfamiliar), then ask again, "What does the card say? Please, read it for us." Ultimately, you can keep the game moving when a player fails to read by moving around behind/beside him/her, so that you are oriented in the same direction as the player: with both of you looking at the index card, as one of you holds it. Be sure to bend your knees so that you are at eye-level with the player. Then, say, "This card says: [reading the card aloud]."

4) **Whether playing by team or individually, the first knick-knack to the top of the pyramid wins the game**. As a result, this game can move quickly, and winning can occur rapidly. I usually recommend several rounds of this game, so that several individuals/teams can be winners.

5) When a knick-knack reaches the top of the pyramid, the "prize" can be as simple as applause or as elaborate as a fresh flower or a prize from a basket of them. It's important to know what prizes are approved by the facility at which one is directing the activity. Some eldercare facilities only permit prizes like stuffed animals, because of the physical risk to individuals with moderate-to-severe dementia who might hurt themselves with a glass object or with an object that has small parts. I often utilize prizes like: paperback books, plush animals, and soft pieces of dietetic chocolate (when approved by nursing staff). Those items are generally safe and appealing to activity participants. For individuals who are normal functioning or who have mild AD, paperback books, paperback word-search or crossword puzzle magazines (with large print), and resin knick-knacks (like those used in the pyramid game) can be excellent prizes. My approach to many games like this one is to provide all players with a "door prize" as they depart, so that the social demand to win the game is reduced and all players leave with a sense of accomplishment (and with a prize to show friends/family).

Activity 2: Wheel of Geography*

Level of Skill: for individuals who are normal functioning and/or those who have mild dementia

Materials: 1 multi-colored pinwheel; 1 poster with tinted envelopes attached; 20-30 index cards with geography trivia questions; and a large rolling-die with a plastic serving tray (the latter, only if using the rolling-die alternative; described below).

"Playing" Time: generally, 30-45 minutes

Preparing Activity Materials:

1) **Buy a multi-colored pinwheel. Attach with tape to its center a white arrow cut from an index card. The arrow specifies the color envelope from which to choose a trivia card.** If funds do not permit purchasing a multi-colored pinwheel, or if

one cannot be located, then make one from stiff cardboard. Simply cut a 9- or 10-inch (diameter) circle from the cardboard and color it (e.g., in quarters, like a pie: red, blue, yellow, white) with brightly-hued permanent markers (or glue on pie-wedge shaped construction pieces). To make a homemade wheel spin, simply punch a hole in the center and use Tinker Toys™ (or similar construction toys) to affix the wheel to a stick. The wheel can be made to stand by sticking it into a foam cup filled with modeling clay or into a large styrofoam (florist's) cylinder. On some occasions, I've made pinwheels that are attached to the lid of a sturdy cardboard box with Tinker Toys™. The box then serves as the "stand" for the display. The "pointer" for the wheel can be as simple as a white arrow cut from a blank index card. Use transparent tape to attach it to the front center (non-spinning piece) of the pinwheel.

ROLLING-DIE ALTERNATIVE TO THE PINWHEEL: If you have no time or inclination to make/find a pinwheel, then try a rolling-die alternative. Get a large set of those fuzzy dice that people hang from their rearview auto mirrors, and snip one of them off the string. Next, cut squares of assorted, tinted construction paper to fit each of the six sides of one die (because one will work just fine for this game). Be sure the tinted squares correspond to the colors of the envelopes on your game poster-board (step #2, below). **Then, use heavy-duty cellophane tape to secure the pieces of tinted paper to the faces of the rolling die.** Be certain that all sides are completely covered with the transparent tape and that there are no loose or sharp edges. When I make one of these die, I "over do" the cellophane tape: wrapping it around-n-around the rolling die, so that there are no exposed paper/cloth edges or surfaces. In effect, the entire die becomes a big, multi-colored "plastic" cube, because it is completely smothered in transparent tape. This makes it easy to wipe the die off with a damp cloth or sponge, so that the group doesn't spread germs through common contact with it.

2) **To construct the poster with multi-colored envelopes is very easy.** Because greeting cards are so readily available, and because their corresponding envelopes come in assorted colors, the chore of finding 4-5 brightly colored envelopes for the trivia poster is easy. I usually build a pinwheel with four colored pie sections. Then, I find four envelopes to match the colors of the pie's sections. If using the rolling-die alternative, then be sure to match envelope colors to the faces of the die. To make the poster, use a glue stick or pieces of transparent tape to attach the envelopes to a poster board. Then, this poster can be hung on the wall (with removable tape, if your facility permits), or it can be made to stand up on a table by attaching a simple folded wedge of stiff poster- or card-board to its back with tape. **When the multi-colored pinwheel is spun, then the color indicated by the arrow is the color of envelope (on the poster) from which the activity leader will choose a trivia question. If using the rolling-die, then it's the color of the die's face after being tossed onto the tray that indicates which color envelope on the poster is to be checked. Be sure to place 8-10 trivia cards in each envelope to support a game of about 20-30 minutes.**

3) Trivia questions can be purchased as card decks at education supply stores, or they can be made by printing simple questions on index cards (with specifications for print size and type given in Chapter 4 of this book). A sample trivia item for geography would be to: "Name a state that is next to Ohio." Correct responses can be printed in small type on the index card reverse, or the activity leader can keep a master list of trivia answers. In this case, Indiana, Pennsylvania, West Virginia, and Kentucky can be given as correct responses. Depending on the level of functioning of participants, one might prefer to make trivia items in question format or in directive format (e.g., "Which states are next to Ohio?").

Question format can work well for normal functioning individuals. However, for individuals who have probable Alzheimer's disease, a question can be daunting. Instead, I find that a simple directive works more effectively (e.g., "Name a city in Florida."). Decide on the format after assessing the needs of your planned participants.

Procedure:

1) I believe that an auditorium-style seating arrangement is best for activities of the type described here. Arrange an activity room with 10-15 chairs in semi-circle formation. If room size doesn't permit just one semi-circle, then arrange remainder chairs in a larger semi-circle as a second row behind the first, and stagger the seats so that those behind can see through the spaces between chairs in the front row. At the front of the semi-circle, place a table. The wheel-of-geography and the poster with trivia cards can be placed on the table.

2) Gather a group of 10-15 individuals who show interest in a trivia or "brain-teasers" game. Some individuals don't like or know the word "trivia", so I call the game "wheel of *geography**brain-teasers*", or merely "wheel of geography". *You'll have deduced by now that this game need not be geography. The trivia cards can pertain to just about any topic you believe might be of interest to your group. Ideas for various trivia games include: state capitals, multiplication tables, history (e.g., presidents of the USA), popular celebrities (being sure to query about celebrities who would be known to the participants based on their ages and preferences, e.g., Frank Sinatra, rather than Tommy Lee for a group of seventy-something ladies and gents!), or famous authors (again being sure to check ages and preferences before fashioning the trivia items).

3a) Begin turns by spinning the wheel. When the arrow indicates a color, then select a trivia card from the envelope of that color.

3b) If using the rolling-die alternative, then begin turns by handing the die to a player. Ask him or her to roll the die onto a plastic serving tray (which you can hold out in front of him/her at the player's waste level—taking care not to hold the tray too high, but instead, low enough for the participant to comfortably toss the die onto it). Then, select a trivia card from the envelope color that corresponds to the color on the top face of the rolled die.

4) Either read the trivia item aloud, or permit audience members to participate in reading (with a participant reading a trivia question aloud at her/his turn).

5) Once a question has been read, then the activity leader can open the floor for answers. In my groups, we usually allow anyone to answer any item. This creates a group effort to participate, and it can make the game much more of a social event. For highly competitive groups, individuals can take turns (by simply starting at one end of the semi-circle and working one's way across it asking questions) and earn points. Know your group and identify which strategy might work best for them.

I used to direct a group on Friday afternoons, and they loved to play the game as a "free-for-all" *with individual scoring*. I'd spin the wheel and choose a question. Then, someone would read the card aloud. After that, anyone could answer, and the player who answered the item correctly and first was the one to get the "point" for that item. At the end of the session, I'd tally the points to let them know who had won the game for that day. The strategy worked very well, and they loved the competition. As one lady put it, "This sort of thing keeps our minds sharp...alert."

That technique with individual scoring did not work well for another group I directed in the evening. They were 7-10 ladies whose cognitive function ranges from normal to moderate dementia. As a group, they are highly cohesive—always helping each other out. A free-for-all did work, but scoring had to be group-oriented. I'd read a question, and whoever knew it would answer. However, they were highly opposed to scoring and very conscientious of others' feelings about measuring up. Thus, for that group, I used the free-for-all technique, but I dispensed with scoring altogether. I'd simply announce at the end of the session which items had stumped everyone. I might say, "Well, it looks like it's time to close up shop for this evening. Thanks for coming out to participate in the trivia game tonight. Wow! The game was great tonight. I believe I only managed to stump y'all on three questions! Be sure to study up on your knowledge about U.S. presidents for next week's game. Well, that's super! Thanks!"

Activity 3: Choose and Win

Level of Skill: moderate-to-severe Alzheimer's and related dementias

Materials: a poster-board with 3-4 envelopes of assorted colors; 1 set of 6-8 prepared index cards for card selection (like "Choose red") with colors corresponding to poster envelope colors; and 1 set of 8-15 index cards for placement in the poster-board's envelopes (with directions for game activities, like "Everyone wins a prize")

"Playing" Time: generally, 20-35 minutes

Preparing Materials:

1) **Prepare a poster-board as in Activity 2.** If a bold heading is printed on the poster-board, then this should be something like "Choose and Win", instead of a title like "Wheel of Trivia" (in Activity 2, above).

2) **Prepare 6-8 index cards to direct color selections.** The print and language should meet the needs of individuals with moderate-to-severe dementia. Use large, bold print (see Chapter 4 of this book). Cards should state things like, "Choose red," "Select blue", "Yellow", or "Pick green". **The color names in the**

statements on the index cards should correspond to the poster-board's envelope colors.

3) Prepare 8-15 index cards for placement in the poster-board envelopes (e.g., one or more cards can go in each envelope). **These cards will indicate what action occurs when a card is taken from an envelope, such as, "Everyone smile," "Win a prize," "Sing your favorite song," "Everyone gets chocolate", "[The activity leader's name] must dance", "Answer a trivia question", or "Wave your arms."** The reader will have noticed that the actions in this game are admittedly simpler than in the previous two activities. It is because of this activity's design for persons with moderate-to-severe dementia. Be sure to have supplemental items available to support the directives on the index cards. For example, at an eldercare facility that permits the activity staff member to deliver snack foods, s/he might have a basket of individually-wrapped chocolate (not hard) candies available for the moment when the "Everyone gets chocolate" card is pulled from an envelope on the poster-board.

Be sure to receive permission from your dietician, director of nursing, or other staff member who oversees elder diets at the facility. Also, be sure to know whether there are participants who require dietetic candy (see Footnote 3, Chapter 4). Moreover, it's best to keep the basket or container of chocolate out of sight (or at least out of reach!) until the chocolate card has been played. Otherwise, a mobile participant with moderate-to-severe dementia might make the entire basket a feast for him/herself! It's also important to un-wrap candies, and hand them to participants by using a food-service glove or by using the wrapper of the candy between your skin and the food. Most participants will reach out to take the candy, and you can gently release it while continuing to hold onto the wrapper. It's an important detail, because persons with moderate-to-severe AD can be so anxious to eat the food that they'll eat a wrapped confection (with the wrapper on!) in seconds—creating unneeded digestive trouble!

If you plan to utilize an index card like, "Answer a trivia item," then be sure to have a stack of trivia cards on hand. I often use state capitals (in the USA) as trivia for Choose-and-Win, because they work well for this game and provide a common, well-known theme for most of our participants. With a more diverse crowd (in terms of countries of origin), the geography theme can be adapted easily to suit their knowledge (like capital cities of nations around the globe: London, England; Paris, France; etc.).

Procedure:

1) Arrange the room in auditorium style seating (as in the above activities). Then, gather a group of 8-10 individuals with moderate-to-severe dementia (with AD and related disorders). If a significant number of attendees will have more severe impairment, then it is wise to utilize two staff members: one to direct the activity and another to attend to participant needs during the game (such as needs for one-on-one assistance with attention, reality orientation, and re-direction from inappropriate behavior).

2) Begin at either end of the group, shuffle the 6 or more index cards with directions to "Choose red," "Select blue," etc. Fan the cards out (as if playing cards) with the blank sides facing up. Then, hold the fan out toward the selected player and say, "Pick a card, any card." Usually, this will prompt a player to comply. If not, it's easy enough to reach for one of the cards, select it, and orient it's printed face so that the player can read it.

3) Once the selected index card is facing the player, then ask, "What does your card say? Please, read it." I find that this task is often difficult for individuals with severe AD during the first couple weeks of playing this game. However, many participants with moderate-to-severe AD do develop card reaching, selecting, holding, and reading aloud over weeks of practice (per the **Six**

Week Rule, I mentioned previously). Even so, for some individuals who have severe cognitive impairments, performance can be unpredictable. Don't fret about it. If a specific player doesn't reach for and select a card, it's easy for the activity leader to select the card, hold it in an orientation so that the player can see it, and even—if necessary—say, "What does your card say? Please, read it. [pausing for 6-10 sec] Choose....What does it say? Choose....[and often the player will interject by reading the color name at this point]...Choose red."

4) Once the card from your hand has been selected and read, then proceed to the poster-board. Select a card from the corresponding envelope (in this example, a red envelope). Say, '[Participant's name] your card said, "Choose red," and the card in our red envelope says, "Sing your favorite song." A word of advice about directing the activity, it's often wise to start the task (e.g., smiling, hand-waving, singing a familiar song) on your own if the player to whom the directive is made is unresponsive to your request. In some of my activity groups, other players will spontaneously chime in, e.g., calling out a song or even starting to sing one when they hear your directive. When singing, it need not involve a song that is begun by the person who selected the card on that turn of the game. It's more important to get a song going and let everyone in the group enjoy the singing of it together!

5) If giving out prizes, then check that they are appropriate for the group you've selected to play Choose-and-Win. Plush animals, small pieces of soft chocolate (again, to dietary specifications), doorknob swags, small wreaths for residents' doors, and books are all prizes that I've given out in this game. As always, the prizes are purchased or made with regard for particular group members' interests and abilities—with considerations about personal safety, too.

6) At the close of the game, it's generally wise to say something like, "Well, it is time for us to end our activity. Thank you so much for participating. I hope you had a good time. I enjoyed it!" and as participants are being transported from the room say, "Thank you, [participant's name]. Thank you for taking part in the game. Have a good [time of day]." All these little things, like thanking people for their time and participation, are part of social decorum. Extending social graces to others is very important for maintaining rapport and for helping others to feel valued—no matter whether their level of functioning is normal or severely impaired. ·

Appendix C

Personal Applications for Caregivers: Taking Respite

What is your worldview? How do you define meaning in life?

For caregivers—whether we are nurse assistants, nurses, adult children of elders who need care, spouse caregivers, or other—long moments become hours and those turn into days. On occasion, the tasks of caregiving can feel unrewarding. Helping with medications, with bathing and grooming, with scheduling and remembering appointments: they are only a few of the many demands on a caregiver. A need for time to reflect is high, but the availability of it is low. Understanding human needs and values is critical for caregivers, because we want to provide high quality care. It's a repeating story for a caregiver to focus on everyone else's needs and ignore his or her own. If we are spent, depressed, and grieving the loss of previous (often better) days, then we might fail when patients, clients, or loved ones depend on us the most!

Re-framing the picture that is your life can be a critical aspect of the caregiver experience. Even if the time is just two hours of respite, it's important to take them just to clear your head! One of my favorite relaxation activities is the hot bath followed by some favorite music. If I can get an hour to detoxify my mind from the whirrrr of chores that keep it so busy, then I can reconnect with my bigger goals. Am I a caregiver? Am I tired? How can I be rested enough to face the next hours, days, or months? *Do not underestimate the power of an hour or two to help pull you back on a course toward good physical (and mental) health.*

Some folks enjoy an evening out with friends. Others like to snuggle into a recliner for an evening with a good book. For a few, the uproar of an exciting football game might be just the right refresher. Know about what rejuvenates you and be deliberate about setting aside time for it. Otherwise, the stress of caregiving might overtake you! Whether it's playing the guitar, watching a baseball game, reading a novel, writing one, or just running as fast and far as you can (only if your health permits it, of course): you know what activities can rebuild your strength. Use those activities as respite and, also, look for the little joys (Brackey, 2003). A shared joke between you and someone for whom you provide care; the song you sing together to celebrate someone's birthday; the time you've spent watching that "big game" together on a Saturday afternoon: these can be savored as high quality moments. They are times that can reduce some of the "lows" of the other minutes in caregiving.

Writing a Personal, Spiritual-Life Narrative

One excellent way to examine different views on aging is to write about personal values and attitudes. What is the meaning of life?

Research on expressive art therapies indicates that creative writing can reduce stress and improve coping outcomes by helping the writer to identify key life themes and interpret them (Pennebaker, 1997). Kaufman and Sexton (2006) reviewed studies of expressive writing and concluded that a narrative format (as opposed to poetry) seems helpful as a route to the "writing cure". If you are writing to vent emotions, process life events, or to "just deal" with things, then try a journal, story-format, or paragraph-by-paragraph composition. I have a friend who carries a journal with her everywhere. When the mood strikes her, she brings it out and starts doodling. She just happens to be one of the most well adjusted people I know!

The two passages that follow are part of my own spiritual-life narrative. My allegories are not intended to provide the reader with definitive answers about the meaning of his/her life. They are just examples of essays—drawn from life experiences and the personal, interpretive narratives that tend to flow from them. As you read my ramblings, think about how you might write, type, paint, or even hum the story of your quest for life's meaning. Throngs of people have lived before us, and many of them have increased in compassion and love for themselves and for others as they've asked and answered life's Big Questions. Does life have meaning? If so, what is that meaning? How do I find the answers to those questions? And how do the answers affect my values, attitudes, and behaviors?

About Life: A Tall (and Short) Tale[1]

In a sunny glen lived a bank of trees. Most of them were mere saplings—offshoots of the roots of their elders. A few of them had lived long, lush lives before succumbing to disease, infestation, or weather. Some of those older trees had fallen and were taking their places in the new order: humus for the nascent generation. On the southwest perimeter stood a terrific oak. It was a tree to drop one's jaw, with strength in its towering stature. One of its roots had run under ground for some six feet and sprouted a sapling. This green, young oak swooshed and swooned under the breezes and drafts of its ancestor.

On a usual day, the old oak wondered, "How great am I? How magnificent is my trunk? It is more than magnificent!"

On that same usual day, the young oak thought, "I am nothing, and it is the fault of that crotchety giant who soaks up all my sun and steals the nutrients from the soil. If that dinosaur would be gone, then I would be able to grow!"

The days lingered on into months in very much the same way: with the old oak in awe of its own prodigious foliage and the sapling longing to be very literally out of the shadow of its predecessor. On a day that seemed very much the same as its antecedents, something different happened when a woodcutter found this verdant paradise.

"This is the perfect wood for my project!" he thought, and he toppled the giant oak, split it into lumber, and hauled it away.

"Finally! I will have my chance!" thought the young oak. However, as the sun dawned bright and hot the next day, the small oak languished. "Oh, the heat! I am parched!" and, later, "Oh, how wrong I was to wish the giant oak away. I will certainly die!" And several days went on this way.

On the tenth day, the woodcutter came back to this spot. As it happened, part of the ancient oak had possessed a twisted, hollowed knot that would be unsuitable for the bench he was making. Indeed, the bench could be all but completed, except for one leg. The woodcutter had been very upset—trying to think about where he might find another fine bit of oak. Then, he'd remembered the younger tree. Now, he'd come back to take it down, too.

"Relief from the sweltering sun!" thought the immature tree as the woodcutter chopped, and then, "But, no. I haven't gotten my chance to become great! Stop!"

The woodcutter hacked the young tree down and carried it off. He used its wood to make the fourth leg of that other tree's nearly-finished bench. It was a magnificent piece of furniture, and so it was that the lives of those two trees in the forest and their lives thereafter were complete and beautiful only as a function of their association: one to the other.

About Life: The Cheese Connection[2]

Big brown eyes were staring at Grampy and waiting for lunch. We sat at the dining room table: Hungry. Over at the counter, Grammy slathered slices of bread with a protective coating of butter, because you "never wanna send a piece of bread out to lunch dry!" She lopped thick, aged Swiss cheese onto each butter-drenched piece, ran them under the broiler, and Voila! We had grilled Swiss sandwiches.

Grampy and I had selected this cheese, especially for lunch, during our trip to the market that morning. Grammy had questioned him, "Bob, I'm not sure that Lauren will eat aged Swiss."

My ten-year-old mind, yearning to connect with grandparents, blurted out, "I love Swiss cheese." And the deal was done. Even though I wasn't at all certain I'd tasted Swiss cheese before, I was committed. Grammy—first reluctant, and now won over by my enthusiasm—bought that package of cheese for us.

As I waited for my sandwich at lunchtime, Grampy asked about my shopping trip. Grammy and I had gone out for bargains, but had we found any? Would we want to look for school clothes tomorrow, too?

And then they arrived in front of us, those two grilled Swiss sandwiches. Grampy's hand went to his forehead. This was his trademark: no folding of hands for him. When he thanked the Lord for a meal, his eyes were shielded!

After a silent moment with eyes closed, he munched his sandwich. Still enthusiastic, I chomped a gigantic portion of the sandwich: Pungent and peculiar. "Aged Swiss definitely has a bite to it," I thought.

To this day, I prefer aged Swiss to all other varieties of cheese. There's no cheddar or baby Swiss for me. Give me the kick of aged Swiss any day, and I remember that special bond with my grampy: to whom, at the age of four I'd announced, "Grampy, you're my best-est friend next to Jesus!"

Human life is about connections, and there are so many ways to construct them. A moment given to another person, your energy devoted to his/her wants and needs, and you make those "cheese connections". Cheese brick by cheese wheel, we build those Gouda times!

About Life: A Commoner's Reaction[3]

There's a juvenile wrestling game that begins with rough-housing. Two children roll around in the dirt, until one player gives-up the game by tapping his/her competitor's shoulder. In the more "spirited" version of the game, the shoulder taps go unnoticed until someone shrieks, "Mercy! Mercy!" This cry signifies a contestant's plea for the game to end—deeming it a lost cause.

When we were young, my sister and I played a "tickling" version of the game. We would roll around and across the densely braided rug in our living room. Because I was very ticklish (markedly so on the bottoms of my feet), it wasn't long before I was laughing hysterically and yelling, "Mercy! Mercy!"

We humans exist in relationships. We wrestle with words, and we tickle each other with compliments. We try to understand other people and their actions. Sometimes we argue, and in our own, many different ways, we cry out for mercy.

Like everybody else, I'm just trying to make sense of things. I also love to read and think and read some more. From my pre-teen years, I'd known that I wanted to go to college and to try for an advanced degree. I wanted to study something with intensity, but my interests were so diverse that I didn't know what to study. I loved biology, art, history, music..., but I had to focus. At the grand ol' age of nineteen, I settled on psychology, with a specialization in human memory research. A moment later I was thirty-five—still dazed and confused—but with middle-aged droop, to boot.

I read books about people who were searching for life's meaning. I wrote a mediocre review article on religiousness in adulthood and aging (Seifert, 2002a). I wrote another about spirituality and creativity (Seifert, 2002b) and co-authored a third about spirituality and religious coping in dementia (Seifert & Baker, 2004). My husband and I took a class on "Understanding God". We concentrated long hours of conversation on poems, the Bible, religion, novels. I emerged from each attempt to understand life even more baffled than I'd been before. By now—if souls have a countenance—mine must look like wet fur on a shivering dog.

Who knows what makes us search? In the fifth century B.C., Confucius suggested that spiritual search denotes maturity. Later, psychologist Carl Jung (1933/1971) seemed to agree. For me, the search seems anything but mature. Maybe it was that cortisol-eliciting, pressure-cooker research career. Maybe it was being electrocuted. Yes: Electrocuted.   Perhaps it was the migraine headaches that crept into my college years and which had now become daily reminders of my imperfection. It might have been my recurring disillusionment with people, who act like they want to love everyone and end up destroying each other out of hatred, greed, jealousy, and selfishness. Whatever the equation, I'd gotten to be thirty-five and thought I was going on two-hundred. I was apt to become that crotchety, bitter character Dana Carvey used to play on SNL who complained about everything with his lips pursed. He was the ultimate stereotype of aging away from "integrity" and toward "despair" (Erikson, 1980).   "I don't waaaaaaant to go outside. The light...<cough, cough>...hurts my eyeeeeeez!"

If spirituality is about the human quest for meaning in reference to the sacred [my paraphrase of Pargament's (1997) definition], then I started my work on this chapter at age thirty-five and at Ground Zero—where meaning seemed gone, because of the absurdity of life and death. When I attended a conference in New York City just weeks after the 9/11 attacks on the World Trade Center, the air was thick and filmy. The profound spiritual weight of the catastrophe was pungent and visible. I'm reminded of Anne Lamott's lament, in her book about the first year of Sam's life: predicting about her son that he will have to know darkness in order to understand light (Lamott, 1993).

Startled and staring through gray air in Times Square, I began to know meaning by believing that I am nothing and something, at the same time. People experience the impression differently. My personal formula was: struggling in my career choices; fighting chronic physical pain; observing with disbelief as calamity killed thousands of people; watching people close to me die from horrifying and painful terminal cancer. Slam! I was face-to-face with a sense of complete and total incapacitation. At the same instant, I began to truly sense the significance of life in space and time.

I'm no philosopher. Thousands of people have reached my conclusion: that each human needs to have a sense of worth. Take that away, and all bets are off. A person who lacks a sense of worth might do anything...or nothing...because, after all, who cares? If life doesn't have meaning, then what does it matter whether we do anything, everything, or nothing?

Religion and spirituality are all about the human "quest" for meaning. We *want there to be a reason for all this, but we can't seem to agree about what the reason is.* This brings me back to the memory of a TV program on which I'd heard a pastor harshly judge Deepak Chopra for not agreeing that Jesus Christ is the one true god who is the one true route to everlasting life (with my apologies that I don't know the minister's name or the program). Synopsis: the minister had figured out life's meaning, and for those who won't accept that one meaning he proclaims damnation. Even if the minister is right, who is he to judge Chopra's soul? Christian Scripture doesn't support his attack on a non-believer. In the New Testament, Christ warned his disciples to "Judge not, lest ye be judged" (Matthew 7:1 NKJV).

So, here I am at a complete stand-still. I believe in God, and I am Christian [and I realize, that this is where the reader might get off this boat: having no patience for a writer who believes in

Christ. If that's true—if you're ready to throw this book out now—*just try to stay with me*, because I have some interesting things to say that don't hinge on your agreement that there is a God who is Christ]. Still, I believe that I am completely inadequate to judge anyone else (per the passage from the Gospel of Matthew referenced above). How can I live? I read Romans 14: 13, "Let us no longer, therefore, pass judgment on one another, but resolve instead never to put a stumbling block or hindrance in the way of another." Thus, I believe I should not judge, because Christ says we shouldn't, but at the same time, Paul tells me in Romans that I shouldn't put a hindrance in the path of another person. Well how can I know whether I'm hindering or helping? Doesn't this take some assessment on my part? And if so, then am I "judging" in a way that I shouldn't? God help me, please.

And this is what it comes to...Your father comes down with Alzheimer's disease and he's told you for years that he "will never go to one of *those places*". Now, you've got to decide whether to place him in a long-term care facility that specializes in caring for individuals with dementia. You know he's said he'd rather die than go to a "nursing home", but he's angry and confused, and he tried to knock your teenage son's head off yesterday. You don't want to go against his wishes. You don't want to *take your father's worth away* by sending him into long-term care. However, you can't manage him at home, and you're afraid that next time he'll really injure you or your son. What do you do? You have to make a judgment.

Or your daughter is being harassed by a classmate, and you seek her teacher's help, only to find out that the teacher couldn't give a flying fruit roll-up and doesn't believe your daughter's story. After all—the teacher has never *seen* the bullying. And it gets worse for a while. Your daughter's teacher actually assigns the bully to a study group *with* your daughter; It's as if the bully has been *promoted.* The teacher seems to be *sanctioning* the harassment!

What do you do? How do you decide whether your daughter is *truly being harassed?* Doesn't that call for some "judgment"? And if you judge, then aren't you going against Christ's directive not to judge? If you're Christian, then that bothers you. At the same time, don't you have obligations to protect your daughter from harm and to teach her how to act with integrity?

Maybe the whole "judge not" directive is superfluous. Plenty of people don't believe in Christ as God and have no use for his advice. If that's you or not, you're still stuck with the dilemma of deciding what's what...of deciding what's right for your life. How do you make those choices? Do you toss a coin? Do you seek the wisdom of friends? Do you ask a numerologist? Do you seek nirvana as Buddha did?

It's especially interesting that a survey of the most widely cited human virtues has claimed both "justice" and "humanity" as the only two (out of six) to be specifically stated across Athenian philosophies, Buddhism, Christianity, Confucian principles, Hinduism, Islam, Judaism, and Taoism (Peterson & Seligman, 2004; Dahlsgaard et al., 2005, Table 2; see this book, Chapter 6). In their handbook of human strengths, Peterson and Seligman stated: "...whereas ...justice lies in impartiality, the virtue of humanity relies on doing more than what is only fair—showing generosity even when an equitable exchange would suffice, kindness even if it cannot ...be returned, and understanding even when punishment is due" (p. 37). It's a profound statement about universal values that these themes of fairness and mercy show up across so many ideologies. People want justice, but we also recognize the need for superceding it in favor of mercy—in favor of humanity.

We can go 'round-n-round' with a debate about philosophies and religions, but we will keep coming back to the same set of questions: 1) Does life have meaning?; 2) What is life's meaning?; 3) How do we find out about the answers to the first two questions [e.g., praying, reading sacred texts, asking friends, watching Oprah, writing to Dear Abby, reading about or doing scientific studies, etc.]?; and 4) How do the answers to the first three questions affect our attitudes, beliefs, and behaviors?

Whether or not you agree with me that there is a God; you're stuck with the same question that I am: Of what to do. By now, if you've made it this far into Appendix C without giving up on me, you're wondering: what does all this have to do with spirituality and aging? It's simply this: that the big questions are the big questions, no matter whether you're two or ninety-two. They're still the big questions whether it's 200 B.C. or 2200 A.D.

When my younger brother was a toddler, he went through a phase (as many children do) of wonderment. He was intrigued by everything, but he was still extremely limited by his own language and cognitive skills. I would say, "Come on. It's time for supper."

He'd ask, "Why?"

I'd reply, "Well, it's been a long time since lunch, and we need food to help our bodies grow."

He'd insist, "But *why?*"

Mom or Dad would chime in with, "A body can't stay healthy without food. Food is what gives us strength."

And he'd become urgent about it, "*WHY?*"

This might go on throughout the meal. Then, we'd go into the evening. Mom would say, "Well, it's time to take a bath and get ready for bed."

He'd ask, "Why?"

...You get the picture....

Like most people, we've been through some stuff. We've lost people who are dear to us; we've had big fights; we've had illnesses. And like many people, we're trying to figure it all out. I'm fortunate to have a loving, supportive family. I'm doubly fortunate to have a husband who has a caring family, too. A couple years ago, my husband said, "I don't think we can ever know 'why'. I'm convinced that the best answer we can get is 'how'." He went on, "OK. So we find out there is a virus that might kill a third of the human race. Virologists start working on techniques to stop the virus from invading human cells by blocking the method the virus uses to attach itself to cell walls. It's about the HOW of the thing. Who knows WHY the virus exists? Who knows WHY the virus attacks humans? We can argue all year about that. One person will decide that it's a judgment from God as punishment for some unclean, sinful human habit. Another person will decide that the virus is just an accident. Yet, a third person will decide that the virus' threat to humans resulted from a logical, observable succession of changes in the virus and in human cells over time. Who's right? Ultimately, does the 'why' affect our virologists? They just need the 'how', so that they can stop the virus from killing all of us."

Then, of course, because I'm me, I ask, "But is it *right* to try to stop the virus? Aren't we making a judgment call when we decide that the virus must be stopped? Isn't that an attempt to address the 'why' question? If I decide the virus must be stopped, then I'm deciding that the human is worth more and the virus is worth less, right?"

Ugh.

So back to the hypothetical about Dad and the long-term care facility. Dad has made it clear to you that he thinks people go to "nursing homes" to die. He doesn't want to go to one, but you can't figure out how to work, keep Dad safe, and keep Dad from knocking your teenager's block off in an argument about whether it's all right for his grandpa to take a walk to the park by himself. Do you need to start asking about the meaning of life? Do you need to ask about why your dad has Alzheimer's? Maybe not, but your actions will reveal your tacit answer to the 'why' question. If you decide that his life can only have meaning if it's on the terms he's laid out for you pre-morbidly, then you'll bend over backwards to keep him at home. If you believe that his life has meaning even if you don't abide by his pre-specified wishes, then you're gonna find a placement for him, right? If you place him in long-term care (or a compromise like daycare), then will you feel guilty? Probably, because his wishes indicate his sense of his own worth. By going against his wishes you've, at least in part, violated his sense of meaning in his life.

According to my husband, we can't know *why*. Maybe he's wrong, or maybe he's not. According to numerous sacred writings, I should not judge. Then, how do I proceed? How do I make wise decisions? Which choice values a father who is ill and keeps a son safe? What option helps a daughter who is being bullied at school?

Not long ago, I watched a film adaptation of Shakespeare's (1600/1923) play, *Merchant of Venice*. Ironically, I saw it on the day I'd begun to rough out this section of the book. There it was: An answer to the question about seeking judgment. We want others to pay for their crimes against us. We want to receive rich rewards, too. In a story about a lender who feels wronged and a borrower who shows disdain for and even negligence with respect to debt repayment, we see realities about human justice. Where the lender seeks revenge, a judge recommends mercy. The twist in human sagas is that we're not nearly as blameless as we'd like to believe. And others are, very often, not nearly as guilty as the claims we make against them.

Shouldn't a lender receive the promised repayment? If repayment isn't forthcoming, then shouldn't the penalty against the borrower be harsh? In Shakespeare's story, set in Venice, Shylock (the lender) begs for fair judgment—without mercy—and receives it. Because he has judged the situation subjectively, he has failed to notice that fair judgment will not lead him to favorable circumstances. Ultimately, he suffers from the penalties of fairness, because he deserves them. The young judge's words surely must ring in everyone's ears. Mercy is closer to God than is fair judgment. We would all be condemned if we depended on justice.

After studying Shakespeare's (1600/1923) play, it seemed happenstance that I turned to the New Testament book of James. Imagine the amazement I experienced when my eyes fell on James 2: 13, "For judgment will be without mercy to anyone who has shown no mercy; mercy triumphs over judgment." It is consistent with Christ's leveling words when onlookers wanted to stone an adulteress; "Let anyone among you who is without sin be the first to throw a stone at her" (John 8: 7 NRSV).[3] I found related advice in Romans 2: 1-2 (NKJV), "Therefore you are inexcusable, O man, whoever you are who judge, for in whatever you judge another you condemn yourself; for you who judge practice the same things."

For the reader who looks to the Torah (Old Testament writings) for guidance, consider the story of Job who was righteous, living with integrity, and who experienced prodigious suffering and loss. A man of God, Elihu, scolded Job for seeking to justify himself. Elihu rebuked, "You say, 'I am in the right before God...How am I better off than if I had sinned?'" (Job 35: 2-3; see Job Chapters 32 - 42). Job suffered greatly and sought justice. He felt as if his own goodness was betrayed. Why try to be a good person if there is no reward for it? Why not just be bad, if one is doomed to suffer anyway?

Elihu's response was: "But you are obsessed with the case of the wicked; judgment and justice seize you" (Job 36: 17). And then, God spoke: "Where were you when I laid the foundation of the earth? Tell me if you have understanding" (Job 38: 4). This story resolves the issue of Job's integrity—of Job's worth—in terms of his relationship to God. In Chapter 42: 2, speaking to God, Job said, "I know that you can do all things, and that no purpose of yours can be thwarted." Finally, Job understood his own worth as a person who was created by God. His worth rested in his relationship to God's supreme wisdom and power.

Carl Jung (1933/1971; 1952/1971), a scholar of great personal conviction, was verbose about the contradiction between a God who is all-knowing, omnipotent, and ever present [e.g., "I am that I am," in Exodus 3:14] and a God who expects to be acknowledged [e.g., by letting Satan test Job's faith]. Ultimately, Jung laid out the power and poetry of the contradiction as the sacrifice of the Almighty to save His fallen creatures. Job's realization was in his value *in relationship to God*; God's sacrifice was in His willingness to become human and suffer in order to save His fallen, human creation—the latter being a most merciful act by a creator who could have just as easily swatted the world into oblivion—as if it were a fly alighting on the back of His hand.

This resolution solves the puzzle of injustice (i.e., Why am I suffering when I am a good person?) in favor of mercy, because a person deserves nothing on his/her own but can be granted mercy (i.e., an unwarranted pardon) and, even grace (an unearned gift). Job stated: "...I despise myself, and repent in dust and ashes" (Job 42: 6). Job's humility and his recognition of his own worth *in relationship to Creation* led God to restore his wealth, health, and social ties beyond their previous abundance.

For the reader who is not Christian or Jewish, the Bible references mentioned here might seem meaningless. They might seem like fairy tales about people who weren't punished when they deserved to be (like the Venetian who didn't repay his debt) or who suffered when they hadn't done anything wrong (like Job). Whether you are religious or not, you might have noticed that people don't always get what they deserve. Some people lie, cheat, steal, or worse. Yet, they seem to get money,

power, fame, and glory. Still other folks work and live with integrity but never seem to get ahead. Your spirituality is your attempt to solve this puzzle. Whether you decide that God exists and that your worth depends on God's mercy; or whether you decide that nothing is real and that your worth is fleeting in every minute; or whether you decide that balance is the only reality and that life's worth occurs as you achieve that balance: Your spirituality will influence your behavior toward others. It will affect your treatment of other people and of the elders for whom you provide care.

Jung (1952/1971) wrote about the ultimate absurdness that an all-wise, ever-present, all-powerful Creator God would ever define him or herself in relationship to mortals (lowly vermin that we are). Jung pointed out, as others had before him, that the solution to the problem is a bridge over the chasm between true perfection and our very real, human feebleness. *What is human purpose except to exist in relationships with others? What is the ultimate purpose of human life except to be in a relationship with the universe?*

Recently, I was shopping for a black, washable blazer. I needed a somewhat sporty jacket to wear at a week-long conference. I found a good possibility on a sale rack at a local department store, and it seemed to fit me. However, I wanted to look around a bit before settling. That was when a petite woman spied the jacket in my possession. "Where did you get that?" she insisted. "Oh, I picked it up right here, " I answered, smilingly indicating the location on the rack from which I'd taken it. She reached for the one in my hands, saying, "What size is this one?" I replied, "Well, it's a 10." Then, fearing that she was about to rip the coat from me, I said, "Uh," and walked quickly to another area of the store with it. Disheveled and stunned, I hurried into the toy section, hoping she wouldn't follow, so that I could think about whether this was the right jacket for me. I bought it for the amazing $8.99 sale price and think it will work well for the trip, but my conscience pangs, "What if she needed a jacket for something *really* important? What if she was scouring the sale merchandise, because she had only $10 in her purse? What if my selfishness kept her from that blazer that she *needed*?" What if, what if, what if? I hope she forgives me for finding it first and not giving it up, and I forgive her apparent aggression (again, my perception). Should I have offered it to her? Perhaps.

Mercy above justice: It's one way to live. In my view, it provides a loophole on the question of meaning if I assume everyone's life has equal meaning, that no one is worth less than I am, and that everyone (including me) should be treated with mercy. Mercy implies the act of giving pardon (and maybe even giving a gift of goodness or graciousness), *despite* what someone deserves. Now, if we could just get everyone to adopt that policy, then murders, rapes, suicides, lying, cheating, and deception would drop-off, right? Nah, that's the justice-seeker's version of the story. The mercy-giver expects nothing, gives mercy, hopes for dispensation, and gives more mercy when equal courtesy isn't offered.

References

Abraham, R. (2005). *When words have lost their meaning Alzheimer's patients communicate through art.* Westport, CT: Praeger.

Adams, P.F., & Benson, V. (1992). Current estimates from the National Health Interview Survey (1991). *Vital and health statistics.* Hyattesville, MD: National Health Statistics.

Adelmann, P.K., & Zajonc, R.B. (1989). Facial efference and the experience of emotion. *Annual Review of Psychology, 40,* 249-280.

Ainlay, S.C., Singleton, Jr., R. & Swigert, V.L. (1992). Aging and religious participation: Reconsidering the effects of health. *Journal for the Scientific Study of Religion, 31,* 175-188.

Aldwin, C.M., & Revenson, T.A. (1987). Does coping help? A reexamination of the relationship between coping and mental health. *Journal of Personality and Social Psychology, 53,* 337-348.

Allport, G.W. (1950). *The individual and his religion.* New York: MacMillan.

American Psychiatric Association. (2000). *Diagnostic and statistical manual of mental disorders.* (4th ed., text revision).Washington, DC: American Psychiatric Association.

American Psychological Association. (1992). Ethical principles of psychologists and code of conduct. *American Psychologist, 47,* 1597-1611.

Arking, R. (1991). *Biology of aging: Observations and principles.* Englewood Cliffs, NJ: Prentice-Hall.

Arroyo-Anllo, E.M., Gil, R., Rosier, M., & Barraquer-Bordas, L. (1999). Procedural learning and neurological disorders. *Revista de Neurologia, 29,* 1246-1267.

Asch, S. (1946). Forming impressions of personality. *Journal of Abnormal and Social Psychology, 41,* 258-290.

Azar, B. (2000, January). Facial expressions: What's in a face? *APA Monitor, 31.* Retrieved May 4, 2004, from http://www.apa.org/monitor/jan00/sc1.html

Azari, N.P., Missimer, J., & Seitz, R.J. (2005). Religious experience and emotion: Evidence for distinctive cognitive neural patterns. *The International Journal for the Psychology of Religion, 15,* 263-281.

Baddeley, A.D. (1997). *Human memory: Theory and practice* (Revised). East Sussex, UK: Psychology Press.

Bahrick, H.P., & Hall, L.K. (2005). The importance of retrieval failures to long-term retention: A metacognitive explanation of the spacing effect. *Journal of Memory and Language, 52,* 566-577.

Baker, M.K. (2005). *Assessing the potential of pantomime as a tool for communication for persons with Alzheimer's disease and related dementias.* Unpublished doctoral dissertation at the University of Akron, Ohio.

Baker, M.K., & Seifert, L.S. (2001). Syntagmatic-paradigmatic reversal in Alzheimer-type dementia. *Clinical Gerontologist, 23,* 65-79.

Barnes, J. (1984). *The complete works of Aristotle: The revised Oxford translation.* Princeton, NJ: Princeton University Press.

Barnes, S., & the Design in Caring Environments Study Group. (2002). The design of caring environments and the quality of life of older people. *Ageing & Society, 22,* 775-789.

Baumeister, R.F., Smart, L., & Boden, J.M. (1996). Relation of threatened egotism to violence and aggression: The dark side of high self-esteem. *Psychological Review, 103,* 5-33.

Bazan-Salazar, E.C. (2005). *Alzheimer's activities that stimulate the mind.* New York: McGraw-Hill.

Bearce, K.H., & Rovee-Collier, C. (2006). Repeated priming increases memory accessibility in infants. *Journal of Experimental Child Psychology, 93,* 357-376.

Beard, G.M. (1874). *Legal responsibility in old age: Based on research into relations of age to work.* New York: Russell's American Steam Printing House.

Beck-Friis, B. (1988). *At home at Baltzargarden.* Orebro, Sweden: Bokforlaget Libris.

Bee, H., & Boyd, D. (2002). *Lifespan development* (3rd ed.). Boston: Allyn & Bacon.

Beland, F., Zunzunegui, M-V., Alvarado, B., Otero, A., & del Ser, T. (2005). Trajectories of cognitive decline and social relations. *Journals of Gerontology: Psychological Science, 60B,* P320-P330.

Bell, V., & Troxel, D. (1997). *The best friends approach to Alzheimer's care.* Baltimore: Health Professions Press.

Bennett, C. (1980). *Nursing home life: What it is and what it could be.* New York: Tiresias Press.

Benson, P.L. (1992). Patterns of religious development in adulthood and adolescence. *Psychology of Religion Newsletter, 17,* 2-9.

Bergman, M. (1971). Hearing and aging: Implications of recent research findings. *Audiology, 10,* 164-171.

Bergman, M., Blumenfeld, V.G., Cascardo, D., Dash, B., Levitt, H., & Margulies, M.K. (1976). Age-related decrement in hearing for speech: Sampling and longitudinal studies. *Journal of Gerontology, 31,* 533-538.

Berk, L.E. (2001). *Development through the lifespan* (2nd ed.). Needham Heights, MA: Allyn & Bacon.

Berkson, G., Andriacchi, T., Sherman, L. (2001). More information on the nature of stereotyped body-rocking. *American Journal on Mental Retardation, 106,* 205-208.

Berridge, K.C., & Robinson, T.E. (2003). Parsing reward. *TRENDS in Neuroscience, 26,* 507-513.

Bianchi, E.C. (1982). *Aging as a spiritual journey.* New York: Crossroad Publishing.

Birditt, K.S., & Fingerman, K.L. (2003). Age and gender differences in adults' descriptions of emotional reactions to interpersonal problems. *Journals of Gerontology: Psychological Sciences, 58B,* P237-P245.

Bitzer, J., & Alder, J. (2003). Sexology for gynecologists. *Gynakologe, 36,* 891-904.

Blumenfeld, V.G., Bergman, M., & Millner, E. (1969). Speech discrimination in an aging population. *Journal of Speech & Hearing Research, 12,* 210-217.

Bolt, M. (2004). *Pursuing human strengths: A positive psychology guide.* New York: Worth.

Bornstein, M.H., & Lamb, M.E. (Eds.). (1999). *Developmental psychology: An advanced textbook.* (4th ed.). Mahwah, NJ: Erlbaum.

Bosworth, H.B., Schaie, K.W., Willis, S.L., Siegler, I.C. (1999). Age and distance to death in the Seattle longitudinal study. *Research on Aging, 21,* 723-738.

Bourgeois, M.S., Camp, C., Rose., M., White, B., Malone, M., & Carr, J. et al. (2003). A comparison of training strategies to enhance use of external aids by a person with dementia. *Journal of Communication Disorders, 36,* 361-378.

Bower, B. (1999, June 12). Elderly show their emotional know-how. *Science News, 155,* 374.

Bowlby, C. (1993). *Therapeutic activities with persons disabled by Alzheimer's disease and related disorders.* Gaithersburg, MD: Aspen.

Bowlby Sifton, C. (2004). *Navigating the Alzheimer's journey: A compass for caregiving.* Baltimore: Health Professions Press.

Brackey, J. (2003). *Creating moments of JOY for the person with Alzheimer's or dementia* (3rd ed.). West Lafayette, IN: Purdue University.

Brewer, E.C. (1898). *Dictionary of phrase and fable.* Philadelphia: Henry Altemus. Retrieved December 28, 2006, from http://www.bartleby.com

Brickman, P., Coates, D., & Janoff-Bulman, R. (1978). Lottery winners and accident victims: Is happiness relative? *Journal of Personality and Social Psychology, 36,* 917-927.

Brownlee, S., & Dattilo, J. (2002). Therapeutic massage as a therapeutic recreation facilitation technique. *Therapeutic Recreation Journal, 4,* 369-381.

Burnfield, J.M., & Powers, C.M. (2006, August). Prediction of slips: An evaluation of utilized coefficient of friction and available slip resistance. *Ergonomics, 49,* 982-995.

Burnfield, J.M., Tsai, Y.-J., & Powers, C.M. (2005). Comparison of utilized coefficient of friction during different walking asks in persons with and without a disability. *Gait and Posture, 22,* 82-88.

Busch, H., & Silver, B. (1994). *Why cats paint: A theory of feline aesthetics.* Berkeley, CA: Ten Speed Press.

Cacioppo, J.T., Hawkley, L.C., Rickett, E.M., & Masi, C.M. (2005). Sociality, spirituality, and meaning making: Chicago Health, Aging, and Social Relations Study. *Review of General Psychology, 9,* 143-155.

Camp, C. (1999). Memory interventions for normal and
    pathological older adults. In R. Schulz, G. Maddox, &
    M.P. Lawton (Eds.), *Annual review of geriatrics and
    gerontology: Vol. 18. Intervention research with older
    adults* (pp. 155-189). New York: Springer.

Camp, C.J., Foss, J.W., O'Hanlon, A.M., & Stevens, A.B. (1996).
    Memory interventions for persons with dementia. *Applied
    Cognitive Psychology, 10,* 193-210.

Campos, J.J., Frankel, C.B., & Camras, L. (2004). On the nature of
    emotion regulation. *Child Development, 75,* 377-394.

Castleman, M., Gallagher-Thompson, D., & Naythons, M. (1999).
    There's still a person in there. New York: Perigree.

Cham, R., & Redfern, M.S. (2002). Changes in gait when
    anticipating slippery floors. *Gait and Posture, 15,* 159-171.

Charles, S.T. (2005). Viewing injustice: Greater emotion
    heterogeneity with age. *Psychology & Aging, 20,* 159-164.

Chow, Y. (2002). The case of an in-home therapeutic recreation
    program for an older adult in a naturally occurring
    retirement community (NORC). *Therapeutic Recreation
    Journal, 36,* 203-212.

Clements, W.M. (1986). Aging and the dimensions of spiritual
    development. In M.C. Hendrickson (Ed.), *The role of the
    church in aging.* New York: Haworth Press.

Cotrell, V., & Schulz, R. (1993). The perspective of the patient with
    Alzheimer's disease: A neglected dimension of dementia
    research. *Gerontologist, 33,* 205-211.

Covanis, A. Stodieck, S.R.G., & Wilkins, A.J. (2004). Treatment of
    photosensitivity. *Epilepsia, 45* (Suppl. 1), 40-45.

Csikszentmihalyi, M. (1990). *Flow: The psychology of optimal
    experience.* New York: HarperCollins.

Dahlsgaard, K., Peterson, C., & Seligman, M.E. (2005). Shared
    virtue: The convergence of valued human strengths across
    culture and history. *Review of General Psychology, 9,* 203-
    213.

Damasio, A. (1999). *The feeling of what happens.* San Diego, CA:
    Harcourt.

Davidoff, J. (1991). *Cognition through color.* Cambridge, MA:
    MIT.

Davidoff, J., & Mitchell, P. (1993). The colour cognition of
    children. *Cognition, 48,* 121-137.

Davis, R. (1989). *My journey into Alzheimer's disease.* Wheaton,
    IL: Tyndale House.

DiGiovanna, A.G. (1994). *Human aging: Biological perspectives.* New York: McGraw-Hill.

Dostoyoevsky, F.M. (1953). *Crime and punishment.* (J. Coulson, Trans.). Oxford: Oxford University Press. (Original work published 1866).

Doty, R.L., Reyes, P.F., & Gregor, T. (1987). Presence of both odor identification and detection deficits in Alzheimer's disease. *Brain Research Bulletin, 18,* 597-600.

Dowling, J.R. (1995). *Keeping busy.* Baltimore: Johns Hopkins.

Drummond, P.D. (1997). Photophobia and autonomic responses to facial pain in migraine. *Brain, 120,* 1857-1864.

Eastwood, J.D., Smilek, D., Merikle, P.M. (2003). Negative facial expression captures attention and disrupts performance. *Perception & Psychophysics, 65,* 352-358.

Ebbinhgaus, H. (1885/1964). *Memory: A contribution to experimental psychology.* New York: Dover Publications. (Trans. H.A. Ruger, C.E. Bussenius, with E.R. Hilgard).

Egloff, B., & Hock, M. (1997). A comparison of two approaches to the assessment of coping styles. *Personality and Individual Differences, 23,* 913-916.

Ekman, P. (1992). Are there basic emotions? *Psychological Review, 99,* 550-553.

Ekman, P. (1994). Strong evidence for universals in facial expressions: A reply to Russell's mistaken critique. *Psychological Bulletin, 115,* 268-287.

Ekman, P. (2003). *Emotions revealed.* New York: Henry Holt & Co.

Elfenbein, H.A., & Ambady, N. (2003). Universal and cultural differences in recognizing emotions. *Current Directions in Psychological Science, 12,* 159-164.

Eliot, T.S. (1935/1991). *Four quartets: Burnt Norton* (Part V). In *Collected poems: 1909-1962.* New York: Harcourt Brace.

Ellis, L. & Ficek, C. (2001). Color preferences according to gender and sexual orientation. *Personality & Individual Differences, 31,* 1375-1379.

Endler, N.S., & Parker, J.D.A. (1990). Multidimensional assessment of coping: A critical evaluation of coping. *Journal of Personality and Social Psychology, 58,* 844-854.

Erikson, E.H. (1980). *Identity and the life cycle.* New York: Norton.

Espinel, C.H. (1996). De Kooning's late colours and forms: Dementia, creativity, and the healing power of art. *Lancet, 347,* 1096-1098.

Field, D. (1998). Special not different: General practitioners' accounts of their care of dying people. *Social Science and Medicine, 9,* 1111-1120.

Fillit, H.M., & Butler, R.N. (Eds.). (1997). *Cognitive decline: Strategies for prevention.* London: Greenwich Medical Media.

Folstein, M.F., Folstein, S.E., & McHugh, P.R. (1975). 'Mini-Mental State': A practical method for grading the cognitive states of patients for the clinician. *Journal of Psychiatric Research, 12,* 196-198.

Fournier, R.R. (1998). The role of spiritual well-being as a resource for coping with stress in bereavement among suicide survivors. (Unpublished doctoral dissertation, Boston College, Boston, 1997). *Dissertation Abstracts International, 59/03,* 956.

Fowler, J. (1981). *Stages of faith.* New York: Harper & Row.

Frankl, V.E. (1984). *Man's search for meaning.* New York: Washington Square Press.

Fredrickson, B.L. (1998). Why are positive emotions good? *Review of General Psychology, 2,* 300-319.

Gallo, J.J., Fulmer, T., Paveza, G.J., & Reichel, W. (2000). *The handbook of geriatric assessment.* Gaithersburg, MD: Aspen.

Galton, F. (1869/1952). *Hereditary genius: An inquiry into its laws and consequences.* New York: Horizon Press.

Gardner, H. (1983). *Frames of mind.* New York: Basic Books.

Garzia, R.P., & Trick, L.R. (1992). Vision in the 90's: The aging eye. *Journal of Optometric Vision Development, 23,* 4-41.

Gibson, E.J. (1969). *Principles of perceptual learning and development.* East Norwalk, CT: Appleton-Century-Crofts.

Gibson, E.J., & Walk, R.D. (1960). The "visual cliff". *Scientific American, 202,* 64-71.

Gibson, J.J. (1966). *The senses considered as perceptual systems.* New York: Houghton Mifflin.

Gitlin, L.N., Winter, L., Dennis, M.P., Corcoran, M., Schinfeld, S., & Hauck, W.W. (2006). A randomized trial of a multicomponent home intervention to reduce functional difficulties in older adults. *Journal of the American Geriatric Society, 54,* 809-816.

Goldsmith, M. (2001a). Through a glass darkly: A dialogue between dementia and faith. *The Journal of Religious Gerontology, 12,* 123-138.

Goldsmith, M. (2001b). When words are no longer necessary. *Journal of Religious Gerontology, 12*, 139-150.

Goldstein, E.B. (2004). *Sensation & perception* (5th ed.). Boston: Brooks/Cole.

Goleman, D. (1995). *Emotional intelligence.* New York: Bantam.

Gordon-Salant, S., & Fitzgibbons, P.J. (1999). Profile of auditory temporal processing in older listeners. *Journal of Speech, Language, & Hearing Research, 42*, 300-311.

Granqvist, P. (2006). On the relation between secular and divine relationships: An emerging attachment perspective and a critique of the "depth" approaches. *The International Journal for the Psychology of Religion, 16*, 1-18.

Grayson, L. (year unknown). [Framed objet d'art with quotation.]. USA: Printwick Papers.

Greenspan, S.J., & Wieder, S. (1998). *The child with special needs: Encouraging intellectual and emotional growth.* (with contributions from Robin Simons). Cambridge, MA: Perseus.

Gregory, R.L. (1966). *Eye and brain.* New York: McGraw-Hill.

Grewal, D., & Salovey, P. (2005). Feeling smart: The science of emotional intelligence. *American Scientist, 93*, 330-339.

Gross, J.J. (1998). The emerging field of emotion regulation: An integrative review. *Review of General Psychology, 2*, 271-299.

Guthrie, J.P., Ash, R.A., & Bendapudi, V. (1995). Additional validity evidence for a measure of morningness. *Journal of Applied Psychology, 80*, 186-190.

Hall, S., Thorns, T., & Oliver, C. (2003). Structural and environmental characteristics of stereotyped behaviors. *American Journal on Mental Retardation, 108*, 391-402.

Hamdy, R.C., Turnbull, J.M., Edwards, J., & Lancaster, M.M. (1998). *Alzheimer's disease: A handbook for caregivers* (3rd ed.). St. Louis, MO: Mosby-Year Book.

Harding, G.F.A., & Jeavons, P.M. (1994). *Photosensitive epilepsy.* London: MacKeith Press.

Hartan, J. (May, 1990). Beyond the patient to the person: Promoting aspects of autonomous functioning in individuals with mild to moderate dementia. *American Journal of Art Therapy, 28*, 99-106.

Hartz, G.W., & Splain, D.M. (1997). *Psychosocial intervention in long-term care: An advanced guide.* New York: Haworth Press.

Hegde, A.L., & Woodson, H. (1999). Effects of light source, illuminance, and hue on visual contrast. *Family and Consumer Sciences Research Journal, 28,* 217-237.

Heider, F. (1958). *The psychology of interpersonal relations.* New York: Wiley.

Hergenhahn, B.R., & Olson, M.H. (1997). *An introduction to theories of learning* (5th ed.). Upper Saddle River, NJ: Simon & Schuster.

Heston, L.L., & White, J.A. (1996). *The vanishing mind: A practical guide to Alzheimer's disease and other dementias* (3rd ed.). New York: W.H. Freeman.

Holahan, C.K., Sears, H.H., & Cronbach, L.J. (1995). *The gifted group in later maturity.* Stanford, CA: Stanford University Press.

Hothersall, D. (2004). *History of psychology* (4th ed.). Boston: McGraw-Hill.

Humphrey, N.K. (1972). Interest and pleasure: Two determinants of a monkey's visual preferences. *Perception, 1,* 395-416.

Hutton, S., Sheppard, L., Rusted, J.M., & Ratner, H.H. (1996). Structuring the acquisition and retrieval environment to facilitate learning in individuals with dementia of the Alzheimer type. *Memory, 4,* 113-130.

Insurance Institute for Highway Safety (2003, March 15). *Status report: Insurance Institute for Highway Safety, 38.* Retrieved June 16, 2004, from http://www.hwysafety.org Keyword "older people".

Isen, A. M., Daubman, K.A., & Nowicki, G.P. (1987). Positive affect facilitates creative problem solving. *Journal of Personality and Social Psychology, 52,* 1122-1131.

Izard, C. E. (1992). Basic emotions, relations among emotions, and emotion-cognition relations. *Psychological Review, 99,* 561-565.

Izard, C.E. (1993). Four systems for emotion activation: Cognitive and noncognitive processes. *Psychological Review, 100,* 68-90.

Janicki, M.P., & Dalton, A.J. (1999). *Dementia, aging, and intellectual abilities.* Philadelphia, PA: Brunner/Mazel of Taylor & Francis.

Jung, C.G. (1930/1971). The stages of life. From *The structure and dynamic of the psyche: Collected works.* In J. Campbell (Ed.), *The portable Jung* (pp. 3-22). New York: Viking/Penguin.

Jung, C.G. (1933/1971). The spiritual problem of modern man. In J. Campbell (Ed.), same edition as above.

Jung, C.G. (1952/1971). Answer to Job. In J. Campbell (Ed.), same edition as above.

Kanouse, D.E., & Hanson, Jr., L.R. (1972). Negativity in evaluations. In E.E. Jones, D.E. Kanouse, H.H. Kelley, R.E. Nisbett, S. Valins, & B. Weiner (Eds.), *Attributions: Perceiving the causes of behavior.* Morristown, NJ: General Learning Press.

Kasteleijn-Nolst Trenite, D.G.A., Guerrini, R., Binnie, C.D., & Genton, P. (2001). Visual sensitivity and epilepsy: A proposed terminology and classification for clinical and EEG phenomenology. *Epilepsia, 42,* 692-701.

Kaufman, J.C., & Sexton, J.D. (2006). Why doesn't the writing cure help poets? *Review of General Psychology, 10,* 268-282.

Kennedy, Q., Mather, M., & Carstensen, L.L. (2004). The role of motivation in the age-related positivity effect in autobiographical memory. *Psychological Science, 15,* 208-214.

Kirasic, K.C. (2004). *Midlife in context.* Boston: McGraw-Hill.

Kitwood, T. (1993). Towards a theory of dementia care: The interpersonal process. *Ageing & Society, 13,* 51-67.

Kitwood, T. (1997). *Dementia reconsidered: The person comes first.* London: Open University Press.

Klein, S.B. (2002). *Learning: Principles and applications* (4th ed.). Boston: McGraw-Hill.

Knopman, D.S., & Nissen, M.J. (1987). Implicit learning in patient's with probable Alzheimer's disease. *Neurology, 37,* 784-788.

Knowlton, B.J., Mangels, J.A., & Squire, L.R. (1996). A neostriatal habit learning system in humans. *Science, 273,* 1399-1402.

Koenig, H.G. (1994). *Aging and God.* New York: Haworth Press.

Koffka, K. (1935). *Principles of Gestalt psychology.* New York: Harcourt Brace.

Kolb, B., & Whishaw, I.Q. (2006). *An introduction to brain and behavior* (2nd ed.). New York: Worth.

Koltko-Rivera, M.E. (2006). Rediscovering the later version of Maslow's hierarchy of needs: Self-transcendence and opportunities for theory, research, and unification. *Review of General Psychology, 10,* 302-317.

Kubler-Ross, E. (1982). *Working it through.* New York: Touchstone (Simon & Schuster).

Kunstler, R. (2002). Therapeutic recreation in a naturally occurring retirement community (NORC): Benefiting "aging in place". *Therapeutic Recreation Journal, 36,* 186-202.

Kunzmann, U., & Gruhn, D. (2005). Age differences in emotional reactivity: The sample case of sadness. *Psychology & Aging, 20,* 47-59.

Kunzmann, U., Kupperbusch, C.S., & Levenson, R.W. (2005). Behavioral inhibition and amplification during emotional arousal: A comparison of two age groups. *Psychology & Aging, 20,* 144-158.

Labouvie-Vief, G., DeVoe, M., & Bulka, D. (1989). Speaking about feelings: Conceptions of emotion across the life span. *Psychology & Aging, 3,* 425-437.

Lamott, A. (1993). *Operating instructions: A journal of my son's first year.* New York: Pantheon Books.

Landauer, T.K., & Bjork, R.A. (1978). Optimum rehearsal patterns and name learning. In M.M. Gruneberg, P.E., Morris, & R.N. Sykes (Eds.), *Practical aspects of memory* (pp. 625-632). London: Academic Press.

Lawton, M.P. (1997). Assessing quality of life in Alzheimer disease research. *Alzheimer's disease and associated disorders, 11*(Suppl. 6), 91-99.

Lazarus, R.S., & Folkman, S. (1984). *Stress, appraisal, and coping.* New York: Springer.

Lehman, H.C. (1953). *Age and achievement.* Princeton, NJ: Princeton University Press/American Philosophical Society.

Lehman, H.C. (1966). The most creative years of engineers and other technologists. *Journal of Genetic Psychology, 108,* 263-270.

Leininger, M.M., & McFarland, M.R. (2006). *Culture care diversity and universality: A worldwide nursing theory* (2nd ed.). Sadbury, MA: Jones & Bartlett.

Leniger, T., Isbruch, K., von den Driesch, S., Diener, H.C., & Hufnagel, A. (2001). Seizure-associated headache in epilepsy. *Epilepsia, 42,* 1176-1179.

Lindauer, M.S. (2003). *Aging, creativity, and art: A positive perspective on late-life development.* New York: Kluwer Academic/Plenum.

Lockenhoff, C.E., & Carstensen, L.L. (2004). Socioemotional selectivity theory, aging, and health: The increasingly delicate balance between regulating emotions and making tough choices. *Journal of Personality, 72,* 1395-1424.

Ludeman, K. (1981). The sexuality of the older person: Review of the literature. *Gerontologist, 21,* 203-208.

Lyubomirsky, S., Sheldon, K.M., & Schkade, D. (2005). Pursuing happiness: The architecture of sustainable change. *Review of General Psychology, 9,* 111-131.

Maas, M., Buckwalter, K.C., & Hardy, M.A. (Eds.). (1991). *Nursing diagnoses and interventions for the elderly.* Redwood City, CA: Addison-Wesley.

Mace, N. L. (Ed.). (1990). *Dementia care: Patient, family, and community.* Baltimore: Johns Hopkins.

Mace, N.L. & Rabins, P.V. (1991). *The 36-hour day* (revised edition). Baltimore: Johns Hopkins (revised version by Warner Books).

MacKinlay, E. (2001). Understanding the ageing process: A developmental perspective of the psychosocial and spiritual dimensions. *The Journal of Religious Gerontology, 12,* 111-122.

Manning, D. (1991). *The grieving reaction: Continuing care series* (Book 2). Hereford, TX: In-Sight Books.

Marshall, B.L. (2006). The new virility: Viagra^{TM}, male aging and sexual function. *Sexualities, 9,* 345-362.

Maslow, A.H. (1966). *The psychology of science: A reconnaissance.* South Bend, IN: Gateway Editions.

Maslow, A. H. (1970). *Motivation and personality* (2nd ed.). New York: Harper/Row.

Mather, J., Stare, C., & Breinin, S. (1971). Color preferences in a geriatric population. *Gerontologist, 11,* 311-313.

Mather, M., & Carstensen, L.L. (2005). Aging and motivated cognition: The positivity effect in attention and memory. *Trends in Cognitive Sciences, 9,* 496-502.

May, C.P., Hasher, L., & Foong, N. (2005). Implicit memory, age, and time of day: Paradoxical priming effects. *Psychological Science, 16,* 96-100.

Mayer, R., & Darby, S.J. (1991). Does a mirror deter wandering in demented older people? *International Journal of Geriatric Psychiatry, 6,* 607-609.

McCrae, R.R., Arenberg, D., & Costa, Jr., P.T. (1987). Declines in divergent thinking with age: Cross-cultural, longitudinal, and cross-segmental analyses. *Psychology & Aging, 2,* 130-137.

McCrae, R.R., & Costa, Jr., P.T. (1986). Personality, coping, and coping effectiveness in an adult sample. *Journal of Personality, 54,* 385-405.

McFadden, S.H. (1996). Religion, spirituality, and aging. In J.E. Birren & K.W. Schaie (Eds.), *Handbook of the psychology of aging* (4th ed.). San Diego, CA: Academic Press.

McManus, I.C., Jones, A.L., & Cottrell, J. (1981). The aesthetics of colour. *Perception, 10,* 651-666.

Meston, C.M. (1997). Aging and sexuality. *Western Journal of Medicine, 167,* 285-290.

Moberg, D. (1953). Church membership and personal adjustment in old age. *Journal of Gerontology, 8,* 207-211.

Moore, T. (1992). *Care of the soul.* New York: HarperCollins.

Morgan, D.G., & Stewart, N.J. (2000). Theory building through mixed-method evaluation of a dementia special care unit. *Research in Nursing & Health, 25,* 479-488.

Musgrave, C. (1997). The near-death experience: A study of spiritual transformation. *Journal of Near-Death Studies, 15,* 187-201.

National Institute on Aging/National Institutes of Health. (1996). *Alzheimer's disease: Unraveling the mystery,* NIH Publication #96-3782.

Nelson, J. (2002, November/December). Spiritual expressions in the caring environment of adult day care centers. *The ABNF Journal,* 136-139.

Nietzsche, F. (1883/1967). *Also sprach Zarathustra.* ("Thus spake Zarathustra": T. Common, English Trans.). New York: Heritage Press.

Olds, J., & Milner, P. (1954). Positive reinforcement produced by electrical stimulation of the septal area and other regions of rat brain. *Journal of Comparative and Physiological Psychology, 47,* 419-427.

Ong, A.D., & Bergeman, C.S. (2004). The complexity of emotions in later life. *Journal of Gerontology: Psychological Science, 59B,* P117-P122.

Paloutzian, R.G. (1996). *Invitation to the psychology of religion* (2nd ed.). Boston, MA: Allyn & Bacon.

Paloutzian, R.G., & Ellison, C.W. (1982). Loneliness, spiritual well-being, and quality of life. In A. Peplau & D. Perlman (Eds.), *Loneliness: A sourcebook of current theory, research and therapy.* New York: Wiley.

Panksepp, J. (1992). A critical role for "affective neuroscience" in resolving what is basic about basic emotions. *Psychological Review, 99,* 554-560.

Pargament, K.I. (1997). *The psychology of religion and coping.* New York: Guilford Press.

Pargament, K.I. (1999). The psychology of religion and spirituality? Yes and no. *The International Journal for the Psychology of Religion, 9,* 3-16.

Pargament, K.I., & Ano, G.G. (2004). Empirical advances in the psychology of religion and coping. In K.W. Schaie, N. Krause, & A. Booth (Eds.), *Religious influences on health and well-being in the elderly* (pp. 114-140). New York: Springer.

Passini, R., Pigot, H., Rainville, C., & Tetreault, M.-H. (2000). Wayfinding in a nursing home for advanced dementia of the Alzheimer's-type. *Environment & Behavior, 32,* 684-710.

Pennebaker, J.W. (1997). Writing about emotional experiences as a therapeutic process. *Psychological Science, 8,* 162-166.

Percival, J. (2002). Domestic spaces: Uses and meanings in the daily lives of older people. *Ageing & Society, 22,* 729-749.

Peterson, C., & Seligman, M.E.P. (2004). *Character strengths and virtues: A handbook and classification.* New York: Oxford University Press.

Phillips, Jr., J.L. (1981). *Piaget's theory: A primer.* San Francisco: W.H. Freeman.

Piaget, J. (1969). *The psychology of the child.* (H. Weaver, Trans.). New York: Basic Books. (Original work published 1966).

Pickford, R.W. (1972). *Psychology and visual aesthetics.* London: Hutchinson.

Pinel, J.P.J. (2003). *Biopsychology* (5th ed.). Boston: Alynn & Bacon.

Plate, S. B. (Ed.). (2002). *Religion, art, & visual culture.* New York: Palgrave.

Poe, (Baker) M.K., & Seifert, L.S. (1997). Implicit and explicit tests: Evidence for dissociable motor skills in probable Alzheimer's dementia. *Perceptual and Motor Skills, 85,* 631-634. [Also, see the *erratum* for Poe & Seifert, 1997, in Footnote 10, for Chapter 2 of this volume.]

Post, S.G. (1998). A moral case for nonreductive physicalism. In W.S. Brown, N. Murphy, & H.N. Malony (Eds.), *Whatever happened to the soul?* Minneapolis, MN: Augsburg Fortress.

Post, S.G. (2001). Comments on research in the social sciences: A more humble approach. *Aging & Mental Health, 5*(Suppl. 1), S17-S19.

Proust, M. (1981). *Remembrance of things past.* (C.K. Scott Moncrief & T. Kilmartin, Trans.). New York: Vintage Books/Random House. (Original work published 1954).

Publius Syrus. (42 B.C./2000). Maxim 557. In J. Bartlett (Ed.), *Familiar quotations* (10th ed.). Rev. by N.H. Dole. Retrieved December, 28, 2006, from http://www.bartleby.com

Rabbitt, P., Diggle, P., Smith, D., Holland, F., & McInnes, L. (2001). Identifying and separating the effects of practice and cognitive ageing during a large longitudinal study of elderly community residents. *Neuropsychologia, 39,* 532-543.

Rabins, P.V., Fitting, M.D., Eastham, J., & Zabora, J. (1990). Emotional adaptation over time in care-givers for chronically ill elderly people. *Age and Ageing, 19,* 623-627.

Radford, B., & Bartholomew, R. (2001, February). Pokemon contagion: Photosensitive epilepsy or mass psychogenic illness? *Southern Medical Journal, 94,*197-204.

Regnier, V. (1997, February). Breaking the mold in nursing home design. *Design'97,* 26-29.

Reisberg, B., de Leon, J.H., & Crook, T. (1982). The Global Deterioration Scale for assessment of primary degenerative dementia. *American Journal of Psychiatry, 139,* 1136-1139.

Riegel, K.F., & Riegel, R.M. (1972). Development, drop, and death. *Developmental Psychology, 6,* 306-319.

Rizzuto, A-M. (2006). Discussion of Granqvist's article "On the relation between secular and divine relationships: An emerging attachment perspective and a critique of the 'depth' approaches." *The International Journal for the Psychology of Religion, 16,* 19-28.

Ronnlund, M., Nyberg, L., Backman, L., & Nilsson, L.-G. (2005). Stability, growth, and decline in adult life span development of declarative memory: Cross-sectional and longitudinal data from a population-based study. *Psychology & Aging, 20,* 3-18.

Root-Bernstein, R. (1999). Productivity and age. In M.A. Runco & S.R. Pritzker (Eds.), *Encyclopedia of Creativity* (Vol. 2, pp. 457-463). San Diego, CA: Academic Press.

Rosenberg, E.L. (1998). Levels of analysis and the organization of affect. *Review of General Psychology, 2,* 247-270.

Rouleau, I., Salmon, D.P., & Vrbancic, M. (2002). Learning, retention, and generalization of a mirror tracing skill in Alzheimer's disease. *Journal of Clinical and Experimental Neuropsychology, 24,* 239-250.

Routtenberg, A., & Lindy, J. (1965). Effects of the availability of rewarding septal and hypothalamic stimulation on bar-pressing for food under conditions of deprivation. *Journal of Comparative and Physiological Psychology, 60,* 158-161.

Rowe, J.W., & Kahn, R.L. (1998). *Successful aging.* New York: Pantheon.

Runco, M.A., & Pritzker, S.R. (Eds.). (1999). *Encyclopedia of creativity.* San Diego, CA: Academic Press.

Rusted, J., Ratner, H., & Sheppard, L. (1995). When all else fails, we can still make tea: A longitudinal look at activities of daily living in an Alzheimer patient. In R. Campbell & M. Conway (Eds.), *Broken memories.* Oxford: Blackwell.

Rusted, J., & Sheppard, L. (2002). Action-based memory in Alzheimer's disease: A longitudinal look at tea making. *Neurocase, 8,* 111-126.

Ruth, J.E., & Birren, J.E. (1985) Creativity in adulthood and old age: Relations to intelligence, sex and mode of testing. *Behavioral Development, 8,* 99-109.

Salovey, P., & Grewal, D. (2005). The science of emotional intelligence. *Current Directions in Psychological Science, 14,* 281-285.

Salovey, P., Mayer, J.D., Goldman, S., Turvey, C., & Palfai, T. (1995). Emotional attention, clarity, and repair: Exploring emotional intelligence using the Trait Meta-Mood Scale. In J. Pennebaker (Ed.), *Emotion, disclosure, and health* (pp. 125-154). Washington, DC: American Psychological Association.

Santayana, G. (1906/1996). *The life of reason: The phases of human progress* (pt. 1, Ch. 10). As quoted in R. Andrews, M. Biggs, & M. Seidel, et al. (Eds.), *The Columbia world of quotations*. New York: Columbia University Press. Retrieved on December 28, 2006, from http://www.bartleby.com

Savary, L.M., with O'Connor, T.J., Cullen, R.M., & Plummer, D.M. (Eds.). (1969). *Listen to love: Reflections on the seasons of the year*. New York: Regina Press.

Schaie, K.W. (1996). *Intellectual development in aging: The Seattle Longitudinal Study*. New York: Cambridge University Press.

Schaie, K.W. (1997). Normal cognitive development in adulthood. In H.M. Fillit & R.N. Butler (Eds.), *Cognitive decline: Strategies for prevention*. London: Greenwich Medical Media.

Schaie, K.W., & Willis, S. (2002). *Adult development and aging* (5th ed.). Boston: Little, Brown.

Schenck, D. (1999). *Cats in hats: 20 assorted notecards & envelopes*. San Francisco, CA: Chronicle Books.

Seckel, A. (2003). *Days of illusions: Page-a-day calendar for 2004*. New York: Workman. [see the entry for August 31.]

Seifert, L.S. (1997). Activating different representations in permanent memory: Different benefits for pictures and words. *Journal of Experimental Psychology: Learning, Memory, & Cognition, 23*, 1106-1121.

Seifert, L.S. (1998). Structured activities reveal residual function in Alzheimer's-type dementia. *Clinical Gerontologist, 19*, 35-43.

Seifert, L.S. (1999). Charades as cognitive aids for individuals with probable Alzheimer's disease. *Clinical Gerontologist, 20*, 3-14.

Seifert, L.S. (2000). Customized art activities for individuals with Alzheimer-type dementia. *Activities, Adaptation, & Aging, 24*, 65-74.

Seifert, L.S. (2002a). Toward a psychology of religion, spirituality, meaning-search, and aging: Past research and a practical application. *Journal of Adult Development, 9,* 61-70.

Seifert, L.S. (2002b). A proposed role for artists in finding and interpreting the sacred. *National Conference Proceedings: School of Visual Arts National Conference on Liberal Arts and the Education of Artists.* School of Visual Arts: New York.

Seifert, L.S. (2006). Maintained reading aloud from index cards in pAD. Unpublished archival data.

Seifert, L.S., & Baker, M.K. (1998). Procedural skills and art production among individuals with Alzheimer's-type dementia. *Clinical Gerontologist, 20,* 3-14.

Seifert, L.S., & Baker, M.K. (2002). Art and Alzheimer-type dementia: A longitudinal study. *Clinical Gerontologist, 26,* 3-15.

Seifert, L.S. & Baker, M.K. (2004). An individualized approach to religious coping in Alzheimer's disease. *Perspectives on Science and Christian Faith, 56,* 181-188.

Seifert, L.S., Drennan, B.M., & Baker, M.K. (2001). Compositional elements in the art of individuals with Alzheimer-type dementia. *Activities, Adaptation, and Aging, 25,* 95-106.

Seifert, L.S., Drennan, B.M., & Baker, M.K. (2006). Intergenerational pen-pals: Making connections through the arts and children's hearts. *Activities Directors' Quarterly for Alzheimer's & Other Dementia Patients, 7,* 27-41.

Shakepeare, W. (1600/1923). *The merchant of Venice.* In W.L. Phelps (Ed.), same title. New Haven, CT: Yale University Press.

Shand, J.D. (1990). A forty-year follow-up of the religious beliefs and attitudes of a sample of Amherst College grads. In M. Lynn & D. Moberg (Eds.), *Research in the social scientific study of religion* (Vol. 2). Greenwich, CT: JAI Press.

Sheridan, C. (1987). *Failure-free activities for the Alzheimer's patient.* New York: Dell.

Shields, S. A. (2005). The politics of emotion in everyday life: "Appropriate" emotion and claims of identity. *Review of General Psychology, 9,* 3-15.

Shmotkin, D. (2005). Happiness in the face of adversity: Reformulating the dynamic and modular bases of subjective well-being. *Review of General Psychology, 9,* 291-325.

Sife, W. (Ed.). (1998). *After stroke: Enhancing the quality of life.* New York: Haworth Press.

Simonton, D.K. (1984). Creative productivity: A mathematical model. *Developmental Review, 4,* 77-121.

Simonton, D.K. (1990). Creativity and wisdom in aging. In J.E. Birren & K.W. Schaie (Eds.), *Handbook of psychology and aging* (3rd ed., pp. 320-329). New York: Academic Press.

Siri, S., Benaglio, I., Frigerio, A., Binetti, G., & Cappa, S.F. (2001). A brief neuropsychological assessment for the differential diagnosis of frontotemporal dementia and Alzheimer's disease. *European Journal of Neurology, 8,* 125-132.

Snodgrass, J.G., & Vanderwart, M. (1980). A standardized set of 260 pictures: Norms for name agreement, image agreement, familiarity, and complexity. *Journal of Experimental Psychology: Human Learning and Memory, 6,* 174-215.

Spoehr, K.T., & Lehmkuhle, S.W. (1982). *Visual information processing.* San Francisco: W.H. Freeman.

Sternberg, R.J. (1997). *Successful intelligence.* New York: Plume.

Sternberg, R.J. (1998). A balance theory of wisdom. *Review of General Psychology, 2,* 347-365.

Stevens, A.B., King, C.A., & Camp, C.J. (1993). Improving prose memory and social interaction using question asking reading with adult day care clients. *Educational Gerontology, 19,* 651-662.

Still, H. (2005). Short term memory difficulties in children, a practical resource. *Child Language Teaching & Therapy, 21,* 223-225.

Szacki, J. (1976, January/March). Social philosophy of Charles Horton Cooley. Originally titled: Spoleczna filozofia Ch. H. Cooleya. (I. Irwin-Zarecka, Trans.). *Kultura i spoleczenstwo, 20,* 79-95.

Szostak, C.M., & Seifert, L.S. (2001). [Sounds that soothe, and sounds that confuse: Multi-modal cueing in probable Alzheimer's disease.] Unpublished raw data. Malone College, Canton, OH.

Tan, R.S. (Ed.). (2005). *Aging men's health: A case-based approach.* New York: Thieme Medical Publishers.

Thomas, W. I., & Thomas, D.S. (1928). *The child in America: Behavior problems and programs.* New York: Knopf. [Reprinted (1970). New York: Johnson Reprint Co.]

Thorndike, E.L. (1898). Animal intelligence: An experimental study of the associative process in animals. *Psychological Review Monograph Supplement, 2,* 1-109. [As cited by Klein, S.B. (2002). *Learning: Principles and applications* (4th ed.). Boston: McGraw-Hill.]

Tolman, E.C. (1959). Principles of purposive behavior. In S. Koch (Ed.), *Psychology: A study of science.* Volume 2, pp. 92-157. New York: McGraw-Hill.

Tomkins, S.S., & McCarter, R. (1964). What and where are the primary affects: Some evidence for a theory. *Perceptual and Motor Skills, 18,* 119-158.

Torrance, E.P. (1977). Creativity and the older adult. *Creative Child & Adult Quarterly, 2,* 136-144.

Tun, P.A. (1998). Fast noisy speech: Age differences in processing rapid speech with background noise. *Psychology & Aging, 13,* 424-434.

Turner, T.J., & Ortony, A. (1992) Basic emotions: Can conflicting criteria converge? *Psychological Review, 99,* 566-571.

U.S. Equal Employment Opportunity Commission. (2003). *Federal laws prohibiting job discrimination: Questions & Answers.* As accessed at http://www.eeoc.gov/facts/qanda.html on June 30, 2003. And see web-site http://www.eeoc.gov/facts/fs-sex.html as accessed on June 22, 2004.

Van Boven, L. (2005). Experientialism, materialism, and the pursuit of happiness. *Review of General Psychology, 9,* 132-142.

Vance, D.E. (2002). Implications of olfactory stimulation in activities for adults with age-related dementia. *Activities, Adaptation, & Aging, 27,* 17-25.

Vance, D.E. (2004). Spiritual activities for adults with Alzheimer's disease: The cognitive components of dementia and religion. In M. Brennan & D. Heiser (Eds.), *Spiritual assessment and intervention with older adults: Current directions and applications* (pp. 109-130). Binghamton, NY: Haworth Pastoral Press.

Vollrath, M., Torgersen, S., & Anaes, R. (1995). Personality as long-term predictor of coping. *Personality and Individual Differences, 18,* 117-125.

Vonsydow, K. (1992). A study on female sexuality in middle and old-age. *Zeitschrift fur Gerontologie, 25,* 105-112.

Vu, M.Q., Weintraub, N., & Rubenstein, L.Z. (2005, May/June). Falls in the nursing home: Are they preventable? *Journal of the American Medical Directors Association, 6,* S82-S87.

Warner, M.B., Morey, L.C., Finch, J.F., Gunderson, J.G., Skodol, A.E., Sanislow, C.A., et al. (2004). The longitudinal relationship of personality traits and disorders. *Journal of Abnormal Psychology, 113,* 217-227.

Warner, M.L. (2000). *The complete guide to Alzheimer's proofing your home: Revised and updated edition.* West Lafayette, IN: Purdue University Press.

Whitbourne, S.K. (2001). *Adult development & aging: Biopsychosocial perspectives.* New York: John Wiley & Sons.

Whitbourne, S.K. (2002). *The aging individual: Physical and psychological perspectives* (2nd ed.). New York: Springer.

Willcocks, D., Peace, S., & Kellaher, L. (1987). *Private lives in public spaces: A research-based critique of residential life in local authority old people's homes.* London: Tavistock.

Williams, L.M. (2006). An integrative neuroscience model of "significance" processing. *Journal of Integrative Neuroscience, 5,* 1-47.

Willis, S. (1997). Intervening in age-related cognitive decline in late life. In H.M. Fillit & R.N. Butler (Eds.), *Cognitive decline: Strategies for prevention.* London: Greenwich Medical Media.

Wink, P., & Dillon, M. (2002). Spiritual development across the adult life course: Findings from a longitudinal study. *Journal of Adult Development, 9,* 79-94.

Woods, R.T. (2001). Discovering the person with Alzheimer's disease. *Aging & Mental Health, 5*(Suppl. 1), S7-S16.

Wulff, D.M. (1996). The psychology of religion: An overview. In E.P. Shafranske (Ed.), *Religion and the clinical practice of psychology.* Washington, D.C.: American Psychological Association.

Zeisel, J., Silverstein, N.M., Hyde, J., Levkoff, S., Lawton, M.P., & Holmes, W. (2003). Environmental correlates to behavioral health outcomes in Alzheimer's special care units. *The Gerontologist, 43,* 697-711.

Zgola, J.M. (1987). *Doing things.* Baltimore: Johns Hopkins.

Zgola, J.M. (1990). Therapeutic activity. In N.L. Mace (Ed.),
  Dementia care: Patient, family, and community.
  Baltimore: Johns Hopkins.
Zifkin, B.G., & Kasteleijn-Nolst Trenite, D. (2000, September).
  Reflex epilepsy and reflex seizures of the visual system: A
  clinical review. *Epileptic Disorders, 2,* 129-136.
Zukerman, R. (2003). *Eldercare for dummies.* New York: Wiley.

Footnotes

Chapter 1

[1] The delusion is self-disproving, because *each one of us* cannot be worth more than *everyone else.* The impossibility reminds me of a visual illusion that was made famous by M.C. Escher. It's an impossible staircase that seems to descend and ascend at the same time. There is an amusing "cartoon" version of this illusion in Al Seckel's (2003; in the entry for August 31, 2004) "Days of Illusions" calendar. One boy appears to go up the stairs while another boy seems to go up in the *opposite direction*!

[2]Dostoyoevsky's novel, *Crime and Punishment*, recounts the tale of an intellectual young man who is enticed by a belief. His delusion that he has a right to decide the relative worth of another human results in homicide. He judges two women as "worthless" and carries out a plan to murder them. This story reveals a lot about the lengths to which a person might go to rationalize his/her sense of superiority over other people.

[3] When we blame others for their mistakes, we seem to do so by attributing their errors to personality defects. Alternatively, we forgive ourselves for mistakes, and blame external causes, rather than character flaws. This "fundamental attribution error" (as psychologists label it) seems to be part of our overall tendency to value ourselves and discount others (Heider, 1958).

[4] In his chapter about the human soul, Stephen Post (1998) denied dualism in favor of nonreductive physicalism. He stated, "The transcendent and eternal value of each individual remains utterly equal" (p. 211). He described the case of Mrs. G., a woman with dementia, whom he visited in a long-term care facility for some years. In describing her situation of cognitive decline, Post made a plea for "agape" (or selfless, divine) love in our interactions with all people—regardless of their mental, physical, social, ethnic, racial, or other status. This principle is present in many sacred writings including Leviticus 19:18 to "love your neighbor as yourself" and Matthew 19:19 (NIV). [See also, Post's 2001 article on ethics in research on Alzheimer's disease.]

[5] With "institutions" developing through the 1960's and 1970's for more standardized long-term care, Bennett (1980) and others called on eldercare professionals to re-evaluate the hospital-

like facilities that nursing homes had become. While the quality of physical and medical care for seniors had improved through the 1960's and 1970's, the emotional, cognitive, and social lives of residents in long-term care often suffered from the "institutionalization" of eldercare (see Bennett).

[6] Fluent aphasia is a language disturbance typified by grammatical, flowing speech that is often devoid of content or which, at the very least, does not represent the meaning the speaker intended. A person with fluent aphasia might query, "How is your brother's dog?"—using a normal rate of speech with appropriate intonation. However, the utterance is an aphasic one if the speaker's intent was to ask, "How is your husband's leg?" I often experienced this type of discrepancy in conversations with Constance.

Chapter 2

[1] In the next chapter, I will discuss how "sensations" change to become "perceptions" when a person imposes actions and ideas on them.

[2] Thorndike's (1898) classic study reveals something about the lengths to which a hungry feline will go to gain food rewards. Thorndike posited that consequences (like rewards and punishments) are actually *necessary* for instrumental learning, while others have argued that rewards and punishments merely alter one's motivation to *demonstrate* what s/he has learned (Tolman, 1959). Olds and Milner (1954) conducted research indicating the power of the "pleasure center" of the brain to motivate action. Rats with electrodes implanted to stimulate that brain region will go without sleep and food so that they can devote more time to pressing a lever for direct brain stimulation (Olds & Miner; Routtenberg & Lindy, 1965). Newer studies indicate that there are two distinct components associated with reward: 1) incentive value (how much a learner *wants* something), and 2) pleasantness (how much the learner *likes* something). According to Berridge and Robinson (e.g., 2003) these two types of brain system are usually yoked, i.e., desiring *and* finding pleasure in the same things. However, it is possible for the two systems to become disparate, so that a person might seek things that do not provide pleasure (high "wanting" with low "liking") or might fail to seek things that would, indeed, provide pleasure (low "wanting" with higher "liking"; see Berridge & Robinson, 2003). The elegant balance between the brain's

regulation of incentive and pleasure provides the foundation for the principles Thorndike (1898) set forth in his *law of effect.* When he described the role that pleasurable consequences play in increasing the likelihood of future behaviors, he was commenting on the balance between "wants" and "likes". We get something we like, and it increases our incentive to seek that thing again.

[3] Piaget described cognitive development from birth to 2 years as "sensorimotor". In this stage of development (which Piaget broke down into six sub-stages), children learn about the world through their interactions with it—through sensing and acting—as in seeing the bunnies on a crib mobile and reaching up to try to touch them. For additional information about Piaget's theory of human cognitive development, consult his works (e.g., Piaget, 1966/1969) or see comprehensive commentaries (like Phillips, 1981).

[4] That is, the American Psychiatric Association (1994), pediatric code 307.3. For more information about stereo-typed behaviors, see the many articles by Berkson and colleagues (e.g., Berkson, Andriacchi, & Sherman, 2001).

[5] There is an entire sub-discipline of gerontology that relates specifically to the biology of aging. Part of this field deals with changes in sensory systems that occur with aging (e.g., Arking, 1991).

[6] See McManus, Jones, & Cottrell, 1981; Humphrey, 1972; Pickford, 1972; but see also Davidoff, 1991, for a discussion of additional issues related to research on color perception.

[7] My apologies to the reader whose favorite color is yellow. I intend no offense. Research on human color preference indicates that red is the most favored, followed by blue, and then by green (Cohn, 1894; as described by Davidoff, 1991). Also, as an aside, there is some evidence to suggest gender and cross-cultural differences in color preferences in adult populations (Mather, Stare, & Breinin, 1971; Ellis & Ficek, 2001).

[8] There is a history of research from the late twentieth century (which continues in this century) concerning links between lights, flicker, visual displays (e.g., computer monitors, televisions), and neurological phenomena such as migraines and seizures. Harding and Jeavons (1994) published a definitive work which has elevated the topic beyond the so-called "Pokemon hysteria" (see e.g., Radford & Bartholomew, 2001). Research on photic stimulation and brain wave activity has confirmed that some individuals are sensitive to visual flicker (e.g., from lights), that

they experience changes in brain activity correlated with the onset of flicker, and that these occurrences can be correlated with migraine headaches, seizures, and related conditions (see Kasteleijn-Nolst Trenite, Guerrini, Binnie, & Genton, 2001; Zifkin & Kasteleijn-Nolst Trenite, 2000; Covanis, Stodieck, & Wilkins, 2004).

[9] Then Malone College undergraduate, M. Hershberger helped with the earliest pilot tests of this technique during the mid- to late-1990's.

[10] When reading the original work by Poe and Seifert (1997), note the type-setting errors on group labels in Table 1 (p. 634). The groups listed in Table 1 should be "*with probable* Alzheimer's disease" (top) and beneath it, "*without* Alzheimer's disease" (bottom), respectively. Both groups showed savings on relearning in the "no" condition, i.e., when they did not recall seeing the puzzle previously. The only individuals who showed no increase in speed across trials were those *without* Alzheimer's disease *who also* recalled seeing the puzzle previously (with *Mean* = -.029, indicating they were the only participants who evidenced no savings in relearning across trials). Presumably, they were the highest functioning participants who were already at "ceiling" (their fastest) puzzle assembly performance on Trial 1.

[11] See Bornstein and Lamb (1992) or DiGiovanna (1994), who noted that the four basic tastes change little with age and that it is the flavors *besides* sweet, salty, bitter, and sour that modify—due to their dependence on the sense of smell.

[12] Klein (2002) wrote an excellent book for readers who are interested in understanding more about principles of reinforcement and punishment in the psychology of learning.

[13] A principal symptom of Alzheimer's disease is short-term memory impairment. Individuals might ask the same question repeatedly, because they quickly forget the answer. The deficit appears to be related to damage in the brain's "hippocampus"—a structure critical for making new information become more permanent in one's memory (Reisberg, de Leon, & Crook, 1982; Gallo, Fulmer, Paveza, & Reichel, 2000).

[14] I reported a procedure that, for the most part, did not utilize sound. Instead, I relied on non-verbal gestures (Seifert, 1999). However, through several years of testing, I have observed that some charades are much more recognizable to hearing persons when they are paired with sounds, and this can actually make the difference between recognition and failed recognition by

individuals with probable Alzheimer's disease. Among the charades I reported in 1999, I have found that the entire category of "animals" and some of the "actions" (like a vacuum cleaner) yield much better performance from participants when I provide voiced sound effects. To reduce the risk of distraction or confusion, the sound should originate from the same location as the charade (with *one person* acting out the gesture and making the corresponding noise). An interesting aside is that voiced sounds seem to distract, rather than help in the category of "musical instruments", because instruments' noises aren't easily duplicated by a human. As one participant told me, "[You] don't make a very good violin, Honey!"

[15] It is also critical to know your facility or organization's *do's and don'ts,* if you're administering care professionally. Some facilities smile on attempts to "keep it real", while others do not. It's important to know the culture of your workplace, so that you don't step into the abyss of taboo topics. I was once running an activity group at a long-term care facility when a participant made a joke that was chock-full of sexual innuendo. One of the staff overheard and said to her, "Oh, that's you, [resident's name]. You're always making jokes!" The resident, who had moderate dementia of the Alzheimer-type responded, "Well, I always say, 'If you can't have sex, then you can at least talk about it.'" And everyone burst into uproarious laughter. The activity staff at this facility had dealt with a preoccupation with sex (among some of the facility's residents with dementia) by removing the conversational taboo. In so doing, they had made the topic less enticing to key residents who sought attention by raising the topic in conversation in order to "shock" listeners. That brief exchange ended the topic, so that the staff member could then re-direct attention to another topic. Contrast with that exchange, the typical conversations in another group with whom I've worked for many years. They are residents at a residential facility that takes a more conservative approach to the topic of sex. I hazard to guess that the topic of sexual relations *does not* appear in casual conversations. Indeed, I'm guessing it would be grounds for a dismissal from one's job. Thus, it's critical to know the individuals for whom one is providing care and it's absolutely essential to know the culture and rules of one's profession (e.g., APA, 1992) and of one's professional environment. Keep in mind, too, that there are federal guidelines for defining gender-based-harassment and sexual-harassment that provide a framework of do's and don'ts in a person's interactions with co-workers (U.S. EEOC, 2003).

[16] Recent research on happiness in adulthood indicates that those who allocate discretionary financial resources with a plan to 'acquire experiences, instead of material possessions' are generally happier (Van Boven. 2005, p. 140, paraphrased). Perhaps, by extension, elders who devote *time* to building meaningful experiences are happier than those who devote it to acquiring material possessions. My inference about time derives from my assumption that *time is at least as valuable to elders as money, because of its perceived scarcity.*

[17] In a review of work on memory differences between Parkinson's disease, Alzheimer's disease, and other neurodegenerative disorders, Arroyo-Anllo, Gil, Rosier, and Barraquer-Bordas (1999) described evidence for a "double-dissociation" of fact-based "declarative" memories from activity-based "procedural" memories. For individuals with Parkinson's disease, planning and remembering one's plan are often excellent (e.g., deciding to reach out for the book on the nightstand; Knowlton, Mangels, & Squire, 1996), but making one's body enact the plan may be problematic. In Alzheimer's disease, the situation is generally reversed—with diminished ability to remember one's plan, but some automaticity in enacting well-rehearsed behaviors (e.g., with a person unable to describe the steps in brewing a cup of tea, but able to actually do so, if the activity has been practiced often; Rusted, Ratner, & Sheppard, 1995; Rusted & Sheppard, 2002; Rouleau, Salmon, & Vrbancic, 2002).

[18] In 2000, I described the case of an elderly woman who was experiencing disorientation and short-term memory loss due to probable Alzheimer's disease. She responded well to assistance restoring a family heirloom. It was key that I provided structure for the activity and that I was able to provide gentle reminders to keep her "on task" as we worked (Seifert, 2000).

[19] While it is true that social support is generally a positive predictor of health and self-esteem, it is also true that individuals differ widely in their perceptions of their affiliations with others (Cacioppo et al., 2005).

Chapter 3

[1] Despite the fierce debate among scientists about the nature of a link between internal emotional states and one's facial expressions (Ekman, 2003; Ekman, 1992; Panksepp, 1992; Izard,

1992; Izard, 1993; Turner & Ortony, 1992; Campos, Frankel, Camras, 2004), it seems very probable that facial expressions play a critical role in human interactions—even if we aren't quite sure how they do so.

[2] I apologize. Although I "googled" the two quotes, I came up empty on the sources. Thus, I must fail at source attribution here. A related sentiment was expressed by Santayana (1906/1996) when he wrote that, "Old age is as forgetful as youth, and more incorrigible...." My view is that the elder years don't necessarily bring rebellious behavior, so much as they bring us to better understand our own intentions and goals.

[3] Some organizations and eldercare facilities frown on the misuse of terms of endearment. Some facilities have very specific rules about methods by which staff should address members or residents, e.g., using "Mr.", "Miss", or "Mrs." or using an individual's first name. If the reader works for such an organization or facility, then s/he should utilize the protocols that are in place there.

[4] I am *not* suggesting that individuals for whom we provide care should be discouraged from constructive grieving and positive coping following loss. I strongly believe that we should encourage individuals through the grief process (see Seifert & Baker, in press). However, a casual conversation as I stroll to the dining room with a resident for lunch might not be the best time to point out that her husband died recently. Sensitivity to an individual's needs for constructive grieving and for time away from grieving is part of supporting anyone who has experienced loss (Kubler-Ross, 1982).

[5] Earlier, in a paper with Walk (Gibson & Walk, 1960), Eleanor Gibson had taken a much stronger "naturist" position—positing that perception of a visual cliff is essentially inborn. With time and additional experimentation, she began to acquiesce to the notion that there are different levels of "preparation" for the visual cliff challenge. Some infants are initially much less sensitive to the visual cues of the cliff than other infants. This opened a door to the idea that learning does, indeed, play some role in visual perception of depth and distance.

[6] My advice here is meant to be illustrative and general. It *cannot* replace the sound advice of a qualified design consultant regarding the reader's specific design requirements and needs. I cannot accept liability for general advice (given here) that is applied to specific situations.

[7] It's my memory that the founder of the facility, W. Howland, was responsible for the design of the exit. At a later date, another, similar exit was added. It was a plain panel that matched the wall covering in that area (speckled blue paint) and which was flush with the wall (with no visible door frame).

Chapter 4

[1] See Footnote 10, Chapter 2, this volume.

[2] Among the activities designed by me (and with various graduate students/collaborators, like Mindy Baker, Diane Sotnak, and Chris Szostak), a common theme is to encourage reading and action by providing simple printed text that provides easy-to-follow instructions. It is common practice in long-term care to keep records regarding resident participation in the activities offered by a facility. And an outcome of the many years of my activities is that I have archival records of reading behaviors for many individuals with probable Alzheimer's disease. Over the years, I have been asked to provide opinions for facilities about which residents might benefit from activities designed to stimulate thinking and memory. Thus, I have had some input (along with facilities' activity staff and residents' families) about which persons might take part in activity groups. On a day-to-day basis, one resident might not wish to participate or another resident might not feel well. Over time, however, idiosyncrasies in individual attendance equalize, and this has allowed me to observe the same people over many occasions and over several years.

[3] I have mentioned in a previous section of this text that advances in sugar substitutes have resulted in many more choices for "food prizes" of this type. No longer are individuals with diabetes excluded from playing (and winning) a candy prize. Consult your facility or workplace for its guidelines about the use of candy or other foods as rewards or prizes. I am always very careful to check the dietary rules and guidelines for each facility and each participant, so that I am in compliance with the needs of and rules set forth for that person. Also, I have found Bazan-Salazar's (2005) book about art, crafts, games, and activities for individuals with Alzheimer's disease to be helpful (see also, Hartz & Splain, 1997; Dowling, 1995; Zgola, 1987; Sheridan, 1987).

[4] Koffka (1935), who was a proponent of the Gestalt "school" of psychology in Germany (circa World War I), made a

statement that is oft misquoted. It was Aristotle (384 BC– 322BC; Barnes, 1984) who'd said, "The whole is more than the sum of its parts." Koffka revived and revised the idea, stating that "It is more correct to say that the whole is something else than the sum of its parts..." (p.176). His suggestions were: that a whole thing is *different* than the simple sum of its parts, and that an entire thing (whether a person, a visual scene, a symphony, or small group) is not just equivalent to the addition of its components. Indeed, properties emerge from the whole that were not necessarily evident through a consideration of its individual parts. For groups, this means that characteristics develop by way of group interactions. Yet, those traits are not necessarily discernible through analysis of the individuals in that group.

[5] However, the participants were not assigned randomly to reading "practice" and "no-practice" conditions. Thus, the integrity of the "manipulation" of reading practice is weakened by its non-random, incidental nature. See, also, Footnote 2, this chapter.

Chapter 5

[1] An intriguing part of any discussion about emotional facial expressions is the study of Gestalt principles that seem to govern perception of so-called "neutral" faces. Hothersall (2004, p. 214) mentioned the works of Galli and of Arnheim which seem to indicate that neutral faces are perceived as older, sadder, and meaner when eyes are more closely set, when the nose is longer, and when the forehead is shorter. In comparison, a face with higher forehead, with shorter nose, and with wide-set eyes is judged as more youthful and serene. It is even more intriguing that this effect (one related to the amount and direction of "cardioidal strain" on one's head) generalizes to inanimate objects like Volkswagen "Beetles" (Pittenger & Shaw, 1975; as described by Spoehr & Lehmkuhle, 1982). Generally, a young child's head has high, negative cardioidal strain, while the same type of strain on an older adult's head is high, but positive.

[2] Although it is true that an individual's current emotional state can be impacted by affective states (both long, lingering moods and short-lived emotions catalyzed by a person's life events and circumstances) and affective traits (personality characteristics that might predispose one to particular ways of perceiving the world and reacting to it), it is also true that we are social beings who

influence each other's emotions (see Rosenberg, 1998). Rosenberg has described a method for analyzing human affect which names *affective traits* as the most enduring, "pervasive", and "broadest" aspects of human emotional life (see her Table 1, p. 251). *Moods* are then conceptualized as "intermediate" with respect to their interval of duration, "pervasiveness in consciousness", and scope of mental and behavior processes they influence. *Emotions*, then, are the most transient, "least pervasive", and most narrow in the breadth of their impact on mental and behavioral processes (see Rosenberg, p. 251).

[3] Beyond personal affect, Shields (2005) has argued that emotions have a "political" nature. People assess each other with regard to whether their expressed emotions are apropos, whether they are expressed and managed within the rules set-forth by group norms, and whether they are expressed in appropriate "amounts" (not too much or too little). Shields contended that complying with or breaking the rules of emotion politics can have important effects on one's social power and status.

[4] The concept "emotional intelligence" seems to derive from an older notion of "social intelligence" which was put forth by Thorndike (as described by Grewal & Salovey, 2005) in the 1930's. The former term likely dates from Peter Salovey's 1986 doctoral dissertation and is subsumed under Thorndike's [broader] idea of a person's adeptness when interpreting emotions and motivations of self and others and responding to those interpretations (see Grewal & Salovey).

Chapter 6

[1] Paloutzian and Ellison (1979) have used the term "spiritual well-being" to describe aspects of personal well-being that specifically relate to the "search for the sacred" (Pargament, 1999, p. 12). One's spiritual endeavors are presumably devoted to this search. A more broad concept is "subjective well-being", which encompasses the self-in-relation-to-the-sacred and the self-in-relation-to-the-ordinary. Shmotkin (2005) used the latter term in a theory about human quests for happiness.

[2] As an aside, I take mild issue with their derivation of a list of Christian virtues from the works of Thomas Aquinas, without contrasting Aquinian views with Augustinian ones, and—especially—without any references to the New Testament.

[3] This story is fiction. It is of my own invention, and any similarities with other stories are purely coincidental.

Chapter 7

[1] A pseudonym ("false name") is used to protect the participant's identity.

[2] In Table 1 of the published article by Poe and Seifert (1997), the group labels were type-set incorrectly. The first (top) group's label should be "**With** probable Alzheimer's Disease", and the second (bottom) group's label should be (i.e., as "**Without** Alzheimer's Disease"). Sincerest apologies for any confusion this printing mistake might have caused readers. See Footnote 10, Chapter 2, this volume.

Appendix C

[1] The first of these personal essays is from a story of my husband's invention (with my adaptation made with his permission). Ironically, the story emerged during a moment when he and I just couldn't see eye-to-eye on something. He was giving himself a "mental lashing" over it, and I said, "Honey, it's done. It's over. We didn't communicate well enough, and we ended up doing things that the other didn't approve. We've just got to learn from it and move on, right?" As I was speaking, he was hearing me and stopped ruminating. At the same time, a wide-eyed and sort-of-vacuous expression fell across his face. I asked, "What in the world are you thinking?" He told me, "You're right. I can't undo history, so I just wrote a short story in my head." Now, I was amazed at this and asked to hear his tale. Being impressed by the theme, I asked him whether I could incorporate it into this book. I'm glad to report that he said, "Yes." [In addition, this story about trees is fiction and written by my husband and me. Any similarities with other stories are purely coincidental.]

[2] This story about cheese is based on personal events experienced by the current author, and any similarities with other stories are only happenstance.

[3] The third application in Appendix C is a highly personalized account of a struggle to find life's meaning. Unlike most of this book, it is not intended as prose based on scientific inquiry. Instead, it derives from my personal worldview: a

derivation of varied epistemologies. Teachers, administrators, and academicians are advised to apply scrutiny to the application's content. Upon adopting the book as a text, please develop course policies (e.g., about required reading of this section) in light of course goals, the teaching context, and/or sentiments about the narrative's content. Whether this particular application is consistent with one's course goals is a personal choice. I encourage individual teachers to apply careful scrutiny before making the choice to exclude or include it. In general, Bible references are to the New Revised Standard Version. *The Holy Bible* [New Revised Standard Version]. (1989). Nashville, TN: Cokesbury.

Index of Terms

Activities,

applications and examples, 29, 31, 33, 36, 42, 46, 73, 93, 106, 113, 122, 135, 154, 157, 167, 168, 189, 193, 198, 203

for elders with dementia, 29, 31, 36, 42, 93, 106, 113, 135, 154, 159, 168, 189, 198

for elders without cognitive impairment, 31, 93, 135, 193, 203

for groups, 27, 29, 31, 42, 106, 112, 113, 135, 154, 189

of daily living (ADL's), 99

of daily living (instrumental; IADL's), 99

person-centered (individual), 11, 21, 33, 46, 48, 51, 52, 58, 70, 167, 187

Zgola's work, 37, 46, 135

Alzheimer's disease (AD), 29, 37, 42, 47, 50, 54, 56, 67, 73, 80, 89, 93, 106, 113, 118, 121, 130, 154, 156, 167, 168, 189

Alzheimer-type dementia (DAT), 29, 38, 47, 65, 75, 89, 106, 108, 112, 116, 121, 169, see also "AD"

Aphasia,

case description (fluent aphasia), 12

general definition, 12, 243

Art activities,

expressive arts (writing), 203, 204

plastic arts (drawing, painting), 47, 106, 163, 167, 168, 203

Attention,

distractions (reducing them in AD), 37, 41, 44, 93, 120, 121,128, 158, 174, 183, 200, 244

Barriers,

physical environment, 73, 76, 80, 249

Caregiver,

respite, 203

spiritual-life care, 155, 204

Confusion,

distractions (reducing them in AD), 37, 41, 93, 174, 183, 244

Order Your Own Copy of

Chasing Dragonflies
(ISBN 0-9791023-0-8)

Add it to Your Library

Price for quantities of 1 or 2 is $15.95 each
Price for quantities of 3 or 4 is $14.36 each

_____Qty X $15.95   = _____

_____Qty X $14.36   = _____

Shipping $4.00 1st book &

$2 .00 for each additional = _____ (within U.S.)

State Sales Tax   = _____
(*OHIO residents*, please add
   6.25% local sales tax)
TOTAL   =_____
Send a check payable to:

Clove Press LTD
P.O. Box 67008
Cuyahoga Falls, OH 44222

Prices are subject to change without notice.

Name: _____

Institution: _____

Address: _____

City: _____

State/Zip: _____

TEL: _____

E-MAIL: _____

For larger orders contact: customerservice@clovepress.com

PLEASE PHOTOCOPY THIS FORM